STAYING ALIVE IS A LOT OF WORK:

Me and My Cancer

Praise for *Staying Alive Is a Lot of Work: Me and My Cancer*

Professional Reviews

Through beautifully descriptive writing…the reader is given a window into not only the physical challenges of dealing with cancer but also the mental and emotional battles that accompany it. Her optimism shines through, making this memoir a testament to the human spirit's perseverance. With its thoughtful narrative and heartfelt moments, this memoir is both moving and uplifting, offering hope and comfort to readers facing their own struggles. Camalliere's journey reminds us that even in the darkest times, there can be light and moments of joy. It's an excellent read.

– Reviewed by Carol Thompson for Readers' Favorite

Staying Alive is a Lot of Work is a profoundly moving and candid account of one woman's journey through the challenging and transformative experience of being diagnosed and treated for head and neck cancer. Pat Camalliere offers readers an intimate look into the emotional, physical, and psychological toll of the disease, while also providing an inspiring narrative of resilience, determination, and recovery. This book will resonate with cancer survivors and caregivers by offering valuable insights into the journey of healing and the power of perseverance and self-advocacy. Pat Camalliere has created a work that not only educates but also empowers others who may face similar challenges.

– Ashley Heidtmann, Speech Language Pathologist

Camalliere's memoir stands as a testament to her determination…inspiring readers to find strength in life's challenges. But the greatest message is to embrace little joys while keeping one's eye on the big prize, which Camalliere accomplishes. Very highly recommended.

– Reviewed by Asher Syed for Readers' Favorite

Pat Camalliere writes in an honest, approachable style that combines personal views with medical information to create an insightful and poignant read. While reading, I was reminded of my aunt, who also battled cancer, and I found comfort in the shared experiences and emotions portrayed in Camalliere's narrative. The author's voice is kind, straightforward, and humorous.

– Reviewed by Zahid Sheikh for Readers' Favorite

The fact that Camalliere is a singer makes her diagnosis even more ironic and challenging, as she reveals in a memoir packed with thought-provoking insights on the cancer survival process's many requirements. From staging to various procedures and cancer-fighting options, Camalliere invites readers on a struggle to not only battle cancer, but regain her life. Her in-the-moment descriptions are key to understanding both the immediacy of daily challenges and the bigger picture of fighting for survival.

– Reviewed by Diane Donovan, Donovan's Literary Services, Midwest Book Review

Recommendations from Other Writers

You will never read a more detailed, heartfelt, and satisfying account of tackling cancer, You will also learn an incredible amount about the treatments and managing the side effects, the good/bad/ugly, in a way that provides valuable information for both patients and their families facing these challenges. A moving story of determination and a sort of how-to manual all in one.

– Sandra Cavallo Miller, author of *Out of Patients*

Gifted historical mystery author and singer, Pat Camalliere is not afraid to relive her brush with death as she takes us through her journey with cancer. It is one that begins on the stage at Carnegie Hall and ends with not just a reprieve from a dreaded disease, but a new reflection on how she viewed and lived her life. It is a book for anyone facing this disease, written with refreshing honesty, unflinching realism, and subtle depth.

– L. B. Johnson, author of *True Course - Lessons From a Life Aloft*

Camalliere's professional background in medical administration gives her unique insight in how to organize and describe her experience in manageable chunks and clear, frank language. This memoir will be invaluable to other cancer patients and their families and to anyone facing an unexpected personal challenge.

– Ruth Hull Chatlien, author of *Katie, Bar the Door*

What Readers Are Saying

My husband had treatment for tongue cancer in 2011. Our experiences were very much like the author's. I wish I had been able to read this before treatment. It will be very helpful to future patients. Excellent explanations and details.

– Anonymous reader

STAYING ALIVE IS A LOT OF WORK:

Me and My Cancer

By Pat Camalliere

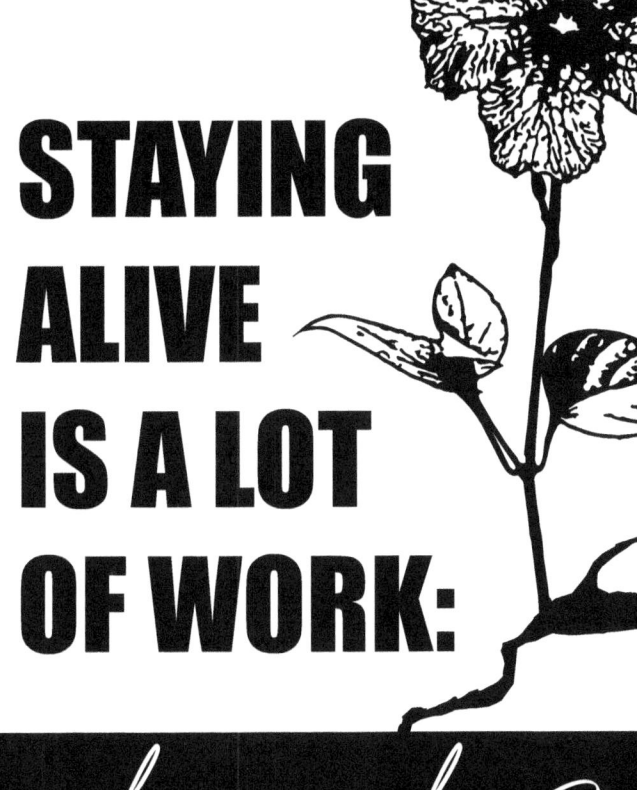

Books by Pat Camalliere:
Staying Alive is a Lot of Work: Me and My Cancer
The Miracle at Assisi Hill
The Mystery at Mount Forest Island
The Mystery at Black Partridge Woods
The Mystery at Sag Bridge

Copyright © 2024, Pat Camalliere

Published in the United States by
Eckhartz Press
Chicago, Illinois

All rights reserved. No part of this publication may be reproduced, distributed, or transmitted in any manner without written permission of the author or the publisher, except for brief quotations as permitted by U.S. copyright law.

This memoir is a truthful recollection of actual events in the author's life. Some conversations have been recreated and/or supplemented. The names and details of some individuals have been changed to respect their privacy.

The author has made every attempt to provide information that is accurate and complete, but this book is not intended as a substitute for professional medical advice. The content of this book is not intended to diagnose, treat, cure, or prevent any condition or disease. Please consult your own physician or healthcare specialist regarding the suggestions and recommendations made in this book. The use of this book implies your acceptance of this disclaimer.

In addition, the publisher and the author assume no responsibility for errors, inaccuracies, omissions, or any other inconsistencies herein. The testimonials and examples provided in this book may not apply to the average reader and are not intended to represent or guarantee that the reader will achieve the same or similar results.

Cover design by Jeff Waggoner. Photography by Pat Camalliere. Designed and typeset by Jeff Waggoner. Edited by Donald G. Evans. Proofread by Lauren Schulz.

ISBN: 979-8-9904639-3-6

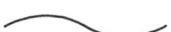

For all those who face serious illness and those who love them.

For all the angels and heroes who provide medical care and compassion.

For all my personal medical angels and heroes, my family, and my friends who were there when I needed them.

Above all to Chris who was with me every step of the way.

PROLOGUE
Carnegie Hall
June 2, 2018

The audience falls silent. The conductor lifts his baton and pauses, capturing the eyes of the tense performers. I take in a full breath—hold it. The baton drops, signaling the downbeat. The orchestra plays two measures, then the chorus begins.

"Kyrie eleison, eleison."

Carnegie Hall, arguably the most prestigious concert hall in the world. The best acoustics in the United States. Where the world's most famous entertainers yearn to perform. Where violinist Jascha Heifetz once replied to a man on the street asking how to get to Carnegie Hall: "Practice." Where I had never dared to dream I would sing.

Yet here I am, on stage at Carnegie Hall.

I am only one in a chorus of almost a hundred singers, ten from the community chorus with which I sing. I stand in the second row near the center of the stage in my black formal dress and look out over the famous rich red plush seats, the tiers of ornate, carved balconies. I find the second tier, first row, left of center, where my husband Chris and son Bob are waving to me. I smile and nod to them, then turn my attention to the complexities of Joseph Haydn's *Mariazeller Messe*, or *Missa Cellensis in C*.

"Kyrie eleison, Kyrie eleison, Kyrie eleison, eleison." Lord, have mercy.

My voice emerges clear and on key, despite my fears that an off-pitch shriek, beyond my control, will emerge from my throat and ruin the program. I breathe a sigh of relief and begin to enjoy the performance.

Singing had been difficult but manageable during rehearsals, when the piece was interrupted frequently to perfect certain sections, and breaks occurred. But here, on stage, is a different matter. The only breaks in the 45-minute work are for brief orchestral or solo interludes. Nor could I sip from a bottle of water or spray my throat in front of an audience. Would my voice hold out? Or would the effects of my cancer have more in store for me?

PART ONE

Facing Cancer

CHAPTER 1
Discovery
November 21, 2017 through November 30, 2017

Two days before Thanksgiving 2017, I found the lump.

The discovery interrupted a near-idyllic time. I no longer had a job or day-to-day responsibility for parents, and my sons, John and Bob, had families and were leading good lives. Chris and I relished the ability to control our own schedules. For the first time in my life, I had free time to engage in whatever activities I chose. I could spoil myself with things that were personally important. I had sung in a concert with the Downers Grove Choral Society earlier that month, and we had just started rehearsals for our next concert in February.

Life was good! The luxury of using my time on *me* seemed too good to be true. But now that the time had arrived, I couldn't shake the feeling of guilt I'd carried all my life. Instead of working on my next novel, shouldn't I be cooking, or cleaning, or volunteering? Doing things Chris wanted to do instead of what I wanted to do? Should I be calling my family or doing some tasks to make their lives easier? What tasks were undone from my responsibilities to the chorus, the library, the historical society? I couldn't get my head around being *entitled* to be selfish.

Newfound freedom had led to my new career as an author. I had successfully published two historical mystery novels and was well into research and early drafts of my third. I knew the craft of writing now; I had a publisher, and I was learning the ins and outs of promoting my books. A lifelong avid reader, it wasn't until after I retired that I mustered up the courage to write a complete manuscript. I had heard horror stories about how hard it was to find a publisher. Instead, I was surprised by how easy it had been and by the popularity I received after my first book was released.

Chris and I would soon be visiting my son Bob, daughter-in-law Dolly, and granddaughter Mia at their home in Fort Wayne, Indiana for a five-day Thanksgiving holiday. John and his wife, Clare, along with my grandsons, Collin and Aidan, would be spending the holiday with Clare's large family this year.

And then, while watching television, I rubbed my neck. I noticed a slightly tender spot under the right side of my jaw. When I pressed the area, I felt a small lump there, about the size of a pea.

I wasn't alarmed at first. *It's that tooth again*, I thought. I'd been to the dentist earlier that same month for a cleaning and exam. He didn't find any problems at the time, although I told him about a troublesome area toward the rear of my right lower jaw. Food collected there between two teeth and my gum got sore, sometimes even inflamed. The lump was right below that spot. I'd had swollen lymph nodes before, years ago when I had some virus, and my jaw had been tender a few times before too. One of those things must be happening. Those other times the problems got better on their own. This will go away too, I told myself.

If it didn't? *Just my luck to come down with something right before a long weekend*, I thought, *when no doctors are available*. At least we would soon be with Bob and Dolly. They were both doctors, not dentists, but I could ask their medical opinion if the lump didn't go away. For almost forty years I'd worked with doctors, and I missed the daily access to personal health care. But having doctors in the family was even better.

I glanced at Chris, who had fallen asleep with the remote control firmly in his right hand, his glasses askew on his face, his bald head reflecting light off the lamp next to his recliner. I didn't want to wake him to mention the lump. Nor did I want to bring up something that could interfere with the planned trip.

The next morning, Chris and I left for Fort Wayne. In the car, I told Chris about the lump, and then I tried to think about the trip and other things. I tried to keep my fingers away from my jaw, but halfway there I gave in and felt the area. The lump was a little larger and a bit more tender. Maybe a food particle got caught between teeth and my gum got infected. Could the tooth be abscessed? Okay, so this might take a few days to get better.

By Thanksgiving Day, the lump was the size of an olive and the muscles on the right side of my neck were sore. I took some reassurance in the fact that I had no fever or other complaints and in fact felt good overall. The lump wasn't painful, only tender to the touch—but clearly something was wrong.

That evening, I told Bob about what I had found, and asked him to check my neck.

Bob took my temperature—which was normal—and felt the lump.

"I bet it's a lymph node that's infected. That tooth right above it bothers me all the time," I said.

"This isn't my field, but that makes sense," Bob, who was a gastroenterologist, said, going along with my self-diagnosis. His voice was calm and professional, and he didn't sound concerned. "I can start you on an antibiotic, just in case. It can't hurt."

By the time we left Fort Wayne to return home on Sunday, the lump was the size of a small plum. Although I was becoming more worried by its size, I still wasn't really alarmed. After all, I still felt good, still didn't have any other symptoms, and it was too soon for the antibiotic to have had any effect.

On Monday, my dentist agreed to see me the same day. A people-pleaser, he was an attractive, boyish-looking man who took personal interest in his patients' lives. After a few minutes spent chatting, he asked what brought me in and then took x-rays of my jaw and did an oral exam.

"Based on what you told me, I thought we'd find an abscess, but your x-ray doesn't show one. I didn't see anything unusual on your exam either. It could still be an abscess though—just too early for it to show on x-ray."

"I think it's gotten a little smaller since I started the antibiotic," I said. I wasn't sure of that, but at least whatever it was had stopped growing.

"I think, based on the history, that you're right, and we're looking at a periodontal infection. I'm going to give you a stronger antibiotic, and it should resolve. Come see me again if it's not better in a couple of days."

Two days later, I had *not* gotten any better. It was hard for me to keep my hands away from the lump. I wanted to keep checking to see if it changed throughout the day. I forced myself not to press on it, thinking that might make it worse.

"Maybe I should see Dr. Earvolino," I said. "Just to be sure there's not something else, something not dental, that's causing this. What do *you* think I should do?" I asked Chris. I still wasn't alarmed, but I didn't want to be stupid either.

Chris agreed. "At our age, it's best to be cautious."

Dr. Earvolino, my internist, worked me into her schedule the following day, November 30. Jennifer Earvolino was a small, pleasant woman with an abundance of thick, brown shoulder-length hair that made me jealous. Her office was at Rush University Medical Center west of downtown Chicago, the same place I worked for fifteen years before I retired, and where most of my doctors were. By then, the lump had been discovered nine days ago. Surely, I thought, she wouldn't find anything. She'd say not to worry, that my dentist was probably right and it would go away with time. I would be happy with that reassurance. That's what I expected.

But that isn't what happened.

"I don't like how this feels," Dr. Earvolino said. "You see Dr. Thomas, right?"

"Yes."

Dr. Thomas was my ENT doctor. I saw him for vertigo and ringing in the ears, which was now better.

"I'm going to see if I can reach him. Stay here." She left the room.

I sat on the end of the exam table and looked at Chris, sitting in a chair across the room. Dr. Earvolino was thorough, one of the reasons we liked her, but surely she was overreacting, I thought. Previous lumps always went away on their own. I was mildly annoyed and made my thoughts known to my husband.

"I'm almost sorry I started this. Dr. Earvolino won't get Dr. Thomas on the phone, and she'll tell me to make an appointment with him. I'll have to wait until one is available and run out to his office—where there's never a parking space—and it's all going to be for nothing, because this is going to go away."

But when Dr. Earvolino returned she looked concerned. "Dr. Thomas agrees. This is suspicious and needs to be checked further. We want you to get a CT scan. And he wants to see you in his office. Can you do that?"

I looked at Chris again. He nodded. He looked worried now. Should *I* be worried?

"We can," I said. "But do I really need all this fuss? I feel fine."

Dr. Earvolino pressed her lips together and raised her eyebrows. I got the point.

"Okay, we'll go. Do you think we can get the scan today, while we're here?"

If I had to get this done, the sooner the better. Better still if we could avoid a return trip. It took from an hour to ninety minutes to get to her office at Rush Medical Center from our home.

"I doubt it," she said. "But let's try."

Luckily, it was still early in the day, and there was an available appointment in an hour. Chris and I walked over to radiology, which was in another building, and I was taken for the scan immediately.

After the scan, we drove home to wait for the result.

"Technicians never tell you anything, just that the doctor will call," I said. "But I'm sure it'll be negative. I feel even better than usual. I have more energy when I should be tired and worried. Wouldn't I feel sick or exhausted if there was something really wrong? And I think it's getting smaller now."

Chris took his eyes from the road and looked at me. "You'd think so," he said.

We were watching television at eight o'clock that night when the phone rang. I jumped up to answer it and took the phone into the kitchen, away from the TV.

"I have the results of your CT scan," Dr. Thomas said. I could hear road noise in the background and realized he must be calling from his car on the way home.

Despite my anxiety, an image of Dr. Thomas came to my mind. A kind and professional-appearing man in his sixties, he was of average height and trim, looking younger than his age, and he always greeted me with a warm smile and a reassuring demeanor.

"Already?" I said. I had expected to wait a few days. My throat went dry, and I felt my face grow warm. *I hope it's good news. Surely it will be good news.* I hovered over the kitchen island, glancing into the family room where Chris was still sitting.

Dr. Thomas cleared his throat. "Yes. I'm afraid it shows enlarged lymph nodes on both sides of your neck. The swelling you feel is invading your neck muscles. It's suspicious. I'd like to examine you in the office tomorrow and take a biopsy."

Tomorrow! So soon!

"Wait," I said. "I want my husband to hear this."

I waved to Chris, who was listening to my side of the conversation from the other room. He came into the kitchen, and I put my phone on speaker. I felt disoriented. Was this happening?

Dr. Thomas repeated what he had told me. Chris touched my arm but looked at the floor, waiting for me to respond.

"Are you saying I have…cancer?" I asked. A tingle like electric current began between my shoulder blades, spread like a wave across my back and down my arms. My hands felt stiff and numb. *Cancer scares me to death, but this doesn't feel real…I'll wake up and laugh in a few minutes.*

When I saw Dr. Thomas in the past, he was cheerful, upbeat, almost jolly, and always made me feel better. Today he seemed different, professionally positive. Through my panicked thoughts, I heard Dr. Thomas say, "We don't know for sure. But whatever happens, rest assured, we have ways to fix this."

A cold sensation surged through my chest—a hint of fear.

He's preparing me for a worst-case scenario…just in case. Or is he? What will Chris do without me? My grandchildren are so young. I want to see them grow up. They need a grandmother to spoil them.

But I said, "Tell me what you're going to do tomorrow." My voice sounded weak but calm.

"An endoscopic exam called a laryngoscopy—insert a thin, flexible tube through your nose so I can look at the back of your throat and tongue. You've had that done before."

"Yes," I said. It had been only mildly uncomfortable.

"We have to know where this started. The CT showed a suspicious area at the base of your tongue, and I want to look at it with the scope. And then we need to find out what that swelling in your neck is. So, I'll numb your neck, put in a tiny needle, drain the lump, and send the fluid to pathology."

"My *tongue*!" I said. "I don't feel anything unusual in my tongue. In fact, I feel entirely fine. This is so unbelievable!"

"Let's hope it all turns out that way. I'll have my secretary call you first thing in the morning to give you a time for tomorrow."

After I disconnected the call, I looked at Chris. I had gotten up that morning expecting to check off a minor health detail. Instead, I had been examined, scanned, and my world turned upside down in a single day.

"This has to be a mistake," I said.

CHAPTER 2
Life Before Cancer: Earliest Memories, 1944-1945

I came from a time and place where mothers stayed home and took care of house and family—housewives, they were called, and it was a profession in those days. My mother was one of those housewives. She grew up on the South Side of Chicago during the Great Depression of 1929-1939 and was married in 1941. World War II started three months later. I was born in 1942.

My father went off to war in 1944, leaving Mom and me behind to live with my widowed grandmother. Leaving his two-year-old daughter and wife without knowing if he would ever return must have been especially difficult for him, as he was a sensitive and emotional Irishman.

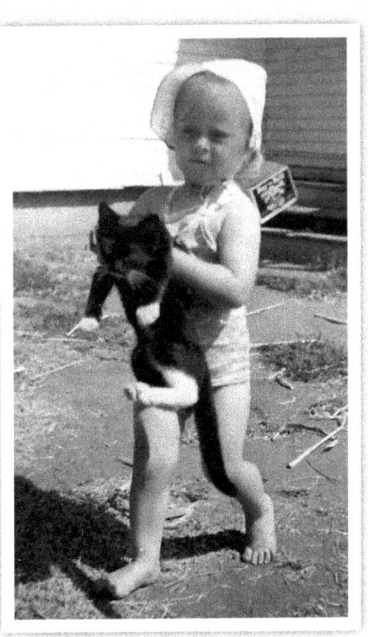

Me, age 2, San Diego farm

Those were not good years. We didn't have much, and we didn't expect much. Our wishes were humble ones. We dreamed only of a modest home and the wherewithal to live a modest life, and that was good enough.

In my earliest memory, my mother and I were lying in a train's sleeper berth. I remember the snug enclosure, being unable to see anything except walls that confined us on all sides, a ceiling mere inches above us. While the train rocked and sped through the night, the rumble and muted "tchjk, tchjk" sound of the wheels on the rails were soothing. I don't remember feeling frightened, or anything, really, except perhaps curiosity.

That memory may have been the first time I became aware of where I was in the world, the first time I wondered how I should react to what was around me. Years later, my mother couldn't remember the incident, but she told me the only train ride she and I ever took was when we went to visit my father in San Diego where he was getting ready to ship out of naval training for World War II. It was our last chance to be with him before he went off to war. I was probably not quite two years old at the time.

In my next memory, Mom and I were walking through tall grass across a field so large I saw nothing in any direction except more grassland—or maybe it was a farmer's field. I wouldn't have known the difference at that age. A tall woman about my mother's age and another little girl near my age were with us. The only thing on my young mind at the time was the speckled gray cardboard suitcase my mother was carrying. The suitcase was tied closed with rope. I wanted to carry it.

"Let me!" I begged, and I cried, and finally my mother set it down and I tried to lift it. And of course, I couldn't, which made me even more furious.

Mom didn't remember that incident either, but she didn't doubt my memory because it fit the circumstances of our arrival in San Diego. We had stayed at a farmhouse with another woman and her daughter near the naval base.

There is no moral or conclusion to this little snippet of memory, but as I recall it so many years later, it may have foretold my spirit of independence, my willingness to tackle the difficult, my persistence, and my tendency to never give up when I wanted something. It also defined me as a person who was strong-willed and wanted to do things herself.

Others who know me now would probably describe these tendencies by another word—stubbornness. I was a good child, but not an easy child.

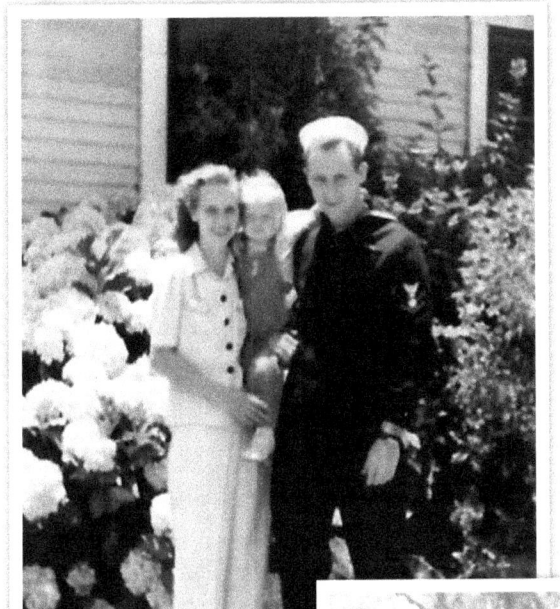

Me with Mom and Dad, San Diego, 1944

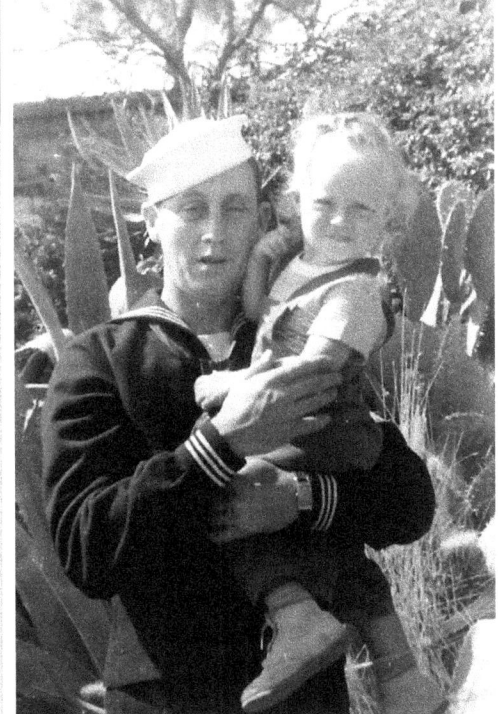

Me with Dad, San Diego, 1944

CHAPTER 3
Results
December 1, 2017 through December 6, 2017

*"I wanted to pray. Nobody in our family ever had cancer.
It was all new to us." – Clare, daughter-in-law*

"I didn't know what to anticipate." – John, son

*"I was afraid. Cancer is a scary word. Was it curable or not curable?"
– Chris, husband*

It wasn't a mistake.

The next afternoon, I sat on the end of an exam table in Dr. Thomas's office.

The doctor sprayed a little anesthetic into my right nostril and throat and a minute or two later he threaded a scope through my nose. The scope, called a flexible fiberoptic laryngoscope, looks like a flexible silver tube, about a foot long, not much thicker than a strand of spaghetti, with a little light on the tip. It is attached to a viewing eyepiece and to a monitor and computer that allows the doctor to view my throat, the back of my tongue, my upper airway, and my vocal cords directly, as well as on the monitor. He can also take and save pictures of what he sees and print them.

Chris sat on a chair near the door, holding my purse on his lap. I knew without looking that he would be gazing at the floor because he was squeamish. I was sure he'd rather be just about anywhere else but would never think of letting me face that day alone.

The laryngoscopy sounds awful, but it really isn't. When Dr. Thomas passed the tube, it felt like some foreign object poking the back of my nose but wasn't painful. As the tube went deeper, there was only mild discomfort. The sensation was a little alarming because it was strange, but it didn't hurt. At the farthest point, the doctor asked me to make an "eeeee" sound. He then withdrew the scope. It was over in about three minutes.

Dr. Thomas set the instrument on a side tabletop and stood where he could see both Chris and me.

"I saw a small lesion at the base of your tongue on the left," he said. "It's in the same area the radiologist identified on your CT scan. About the size of the tip of my little finger." He held up his hand, pinching the tip of his fifth finger with his thumbnail. "Now let's check that lump in your neck."

"It was much bigger," I said, nervously. "It's gone down a lot." In fact, it had gone down a fair amount, but was still about the size of a grape.

Dr. Thomas nodded. He moved to my side and felt behind my ears, down the sides of my neck, under my jaw, and around my voice box. When he anesthetized the area around the lump, I was prepared for significant pain. I closed my eyes. But I felt a little sting when the medication was injected and then nothing at all. I opened my eyes and glanced at Chris. As expected, he was looking at the floor again.

At the right side of my neck, I felt only a slight pressure, but Dr. Thomas told me what he was doing as he inserted a thin needle and withdrew fluid.

"Interesting," he said. "This looks like pus."

I was my father's child, always looking for an opportunity for a funny line, and never more desperately than when something unpleasant was going on.

"Yay!" I said. "Pus!" Then I giggled. For a moment I was relieved. I took the doctor's comment as a good sign. Perhaps pus meant this was an infection and not cancer after all.

My eyes sought out first Chris, then Dr. Thomas, hopefully.

"Let's let the pathologist tell us," Dr. Thomas said.

I closed my eyes again. When finished, he handed a glass tube to a nurse. I thought, *Please, God, let this be an infection!*

At home that night, I called Bob to give him what I thought was an encouraging update. I was disappointed when Bob didn't think the presence of pus was as significant as I did. After feeling responsible for my sons since their birth, it now felt strange to be looking to them for support. Strange, but also appreciative.

"I hope it's not cancer, too, but that would be hard to believe in view of the CT report," he said. "In any case, it's fortunate we have an oncologist in the family. Dolly will be a huge help to you if need be. She'd like to believe it's an infection too, but we're both concerned. We'll get you through this, Mom."

It was a week before Dr. Thomas called with the results of the culture and pathology. This time it was late morning when he called. The report confirmed the presence of infection.

"Unfortunately," he said, "that's not all. Cancer cells were also present."

My heart began to race, and I could feel my cheeks burning. I clutched my phone tightly where I stood in the kitchen. Chris was at the sink. I put the phone on speaker and poked Chris to be sure he was listening.

"What caused the infection?" I asked.

"We can't be sure at this point," Dr. Thomas said. "It could be a dental infection—as you first thought—that was in the process of resolving. Infection is no longer a concern, though."

"But where did the cancer come from?"

"Again, it's too soon to tell for sure, but the most likely cause is the lesion on your tongue."

I was bewildered. "I don't understand...uhm..." I struggled to find the right words. "If the cancer is on the *left* side of the back of my tongue, why were cancer cells found in the lump on the *right* side of my neck?"

He hesitated. I suspected he didn't want to say too much. There must be more bad news to come.

"Remember that the CT scan showed, along with the suspicious lesion on your tongue, that you had enlarged lymph nodes on *both* sides of your neck." He paused. "You're going to need more studies to be sure it hasn't spread to other areas of your neck or elsewhere. We don't know enough yet."

I was stunned. This was alarming. *What? I not only have cancer, but it's already spread? This is bad. Very bad.*

I fought to concentrate on his words.

"Before I called you, we discussed your case at tumor board."

I knew what tumor board was because when I worked at Rush the surgeons I worked with participated in it. Medical oncologists, radiation oncologists, and surgical specialists sat down regularly to discuss every cancer patient being treated. To pick everyone's brain, so to speak, to come to agreement on the best course of treatment and analyze results of treatment in progress.

"It was the board's consensus that we found your cancer early. The prognosis for treatment and cure looks favorable. There's a good chance we can avoid radical surgery, depending on the results of a PET scan and direct biopsy of your tongue lesion. If it all comes out as we believe it will, we may be able to offer you an alternative treatment—a study protocol that will be easier on you and less invasive than standard treatment."

Radical surgery. Biopsy. Study protocol. Favorable? Disoriented again, I fought to understand the words that seemed to be coming too rapidly to digest.

"What would that be like?" I asked, rattling off the question like a robot.

"We would do an open biopsy of the lesion on your tongue under general anesthesia. That would be followed by seven weeks of a combination of radiation therapy and chemotherapy. The study protocol would limit the areas we radiate, and the chemotherapy agent is better tolerated than standard treatment."

I understood medical-speak pretty well, but I wished he'd slow down.

"I wouldn't need a radical neck dissection then?"

Dr. Thomas hadn't mentioned a radical neck dissection, but I knew what that was from working with surgeons. When multiple lymph nodes in the neck were cancerous, it took an extensive seven-hour surgery to remove all the lymph nodes in the neck, teasing them out tediously. The outcome was often disfiguring, and the result was not always good.

I couldn't believe this was happening to me. I felt so healthy! Especially now that the lump in my neck had been drained and responded to antibiotics—it was essentially gone now. My energy level was as good as it had been in a long time. I felt like I could run around the block if I wanted to! This must all be a mistake. Somebody else's report or something. Not me!

"I don't think so, but let's get you set up for that PET scan and an appointment with oncology, then we can answer that question. My office will call you to help make those arrangements."

But I said, "What will happen if I don't treat it? If I do nothing?" Maybe it would go away if I waited awhile, or the mistake would be found. One of the surgeons I worked for liked to use the term "tincture of time." Again, I had that detached, unreal feeling.

"It will spread. There is no ignoring this."

One thing I knew for sure: I wanted to live.

CHAPTER 4
Life Before Cancer: Toddler Years, 1945

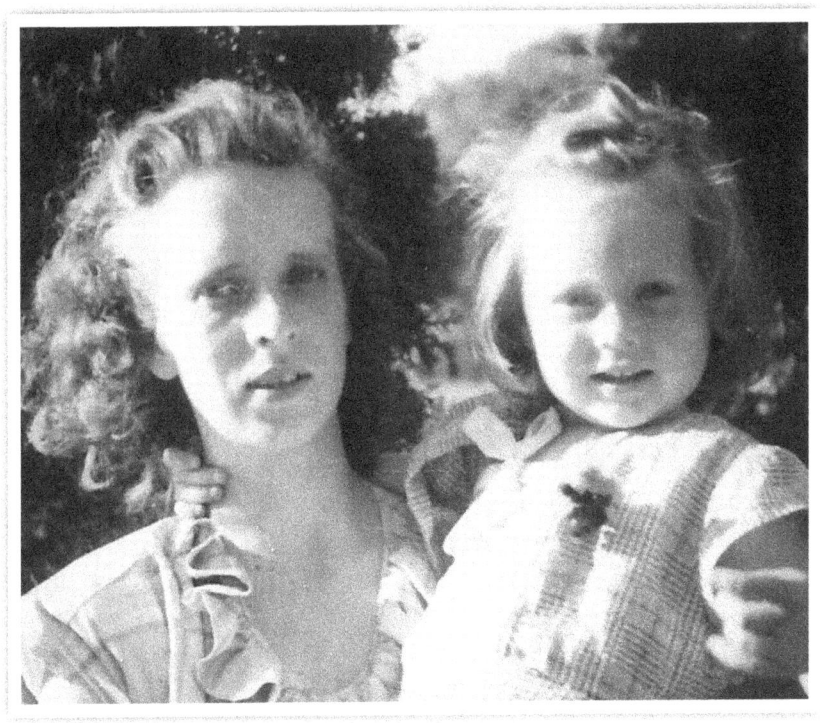

Mom and Me

Another early memory must have happened after we returned from San Diego, because only my mother and my aunt were present. We lived then in a quiet neighborhood on the South Side of Chicago. Grandma lived downstairs in the two-flat she owned, and my single Aunt Isabel and my divorced Uncle Teddy lived with her. My mother and father lived upstairs in the second-floor flat with me, except when Dad was away fighting in World War II. My only brother was not born until years later, when I was eight years old.

During those war years, every morning Grandma woke before everyone else, put on a house dress, long light tan stockings, sturdy black laced shoes, and a beaten-up gray sweater, and went to the coalbin in the basement to "make fire" in the furnace and hot water in the water stove. She made hot water only once in the morning, plus once every Saturday evening for baths. After "making fire," Grandma would walk about a half mile to a factory, where she worked during the war.

Grandma, my mother's mother, was a widow. Although her parents were immigrants, she had been born in Chicago and she spoke Polish as fluently as English. She was educated only through fifth grade. She survived three husbands and her first daughter, Gertrude, who had died in 1910 at the age of two. She raised six children to adulthood. Years later, when she was in her mid-sixties, Grandma had a boyfriend, Steve, who probably would have been husband number four, but this time he died before they were married. He had made her laugh, but Grandma was the only one that liked him. After that, she gave up on men.

Evelyn, my mother, was Grandma's youngest child, yet somehow, I was the oldest grandchild. Grandma was usually too busy to play with me. She was not a warm-mannered person, but she was the strongest, hardest-working, and kindest woman I have ever known. She kept a canary in a cage in her dining room and cared for injured robins and sparrows in another cage on her enclosed back porch. She let me hold the birds now and then, wrapped in a tissue so they wouldn't give me some bird disease.

Grandma also always had a dog, some goofy stray or other that just appeared one day and became part of the household. One I remember was named Buttons, a terrier. No matter how long Grandma left Buttons to roam in the fenced backyard and "do his business," as soon as he got back in the house he would make a beeline for the bathtub, hop in, and do it there. For *some reason Grandma never got into the habit of keeping the bathroom door closed, but that was Grandma. She always called her dogs the same thing, no matter what they were named: That Damn Ky-Yoodle. I never knew what that meant—probably something in Polish. Daddy always laughed when Grandma cussed her dogs, although he was actually very fond of her.*

The dog she owned on that summer day was named Bozo. He was a mean, middle-sized black mongrel who had bitten many people, so Grandma kept him chained up near the basement door. I was terrified of Bozo, but I had to walk near him to get to the yard. As I went down the porch stairs, he would bark and growl and leap against his chain every time.

Despite this, my mother dragged me past Bozo almost every day, weather permitting, to be sure I got regular exercise in our yard. My memory of the yard is clear to this day. It was about twenty-five feet wide and fifty feet deep. On one side was a concrete walk that led from the gangway alongside the house and ended at a gate to an alley that ran behind the house. In summer, hollyhocks grew in the back corner of the yard, with a vegetable garden across the back fence. Opposite the walk was a strip of flower garden that went all the way from the house to the alley. In the center of the lawn was a small bed of roses, and between the roses and the vegetable garden was a large cottonwood poplar tree. My father had made a wooden bench that circled the base of the tree and finished it with shiny dark green paint. I loved that yard.

We lived near Midway Airport, which was Chicago's only airport at that time. As the war was ending, planes would fly low over our yard. On more than one occasion my mother and aunt would wave and cheer as a plane went over. Mom told me those planes were military planes full of men coming home from the war, and that soon my father would be on one of them.

That summer day, after "running the gauntlet" past Bozo, my mother and aunt were working in the garden while I played. After a while, I realized I needed to "pee-pee." I told my mother and aunt they had to take me in to "potty." I remember that I had recently changed to wearing panties instead of diapers and prided myself on never having an accident. But Mommy and Auntie thought I just wanted attention and kept gardening until the inevitable happened and I wet my pants.

"See!" I shouted at them through my frustration and tears. "I told you! Why didn't you believe me?"

The incident must have been traumatic to stick in my mind so many years later. To this day, my expectations are high when it comes to the truth. Nothing makes me more furious than not being believed. If I tell you something, you better not doubt me, or my wrath will be released, likely disproportionately.

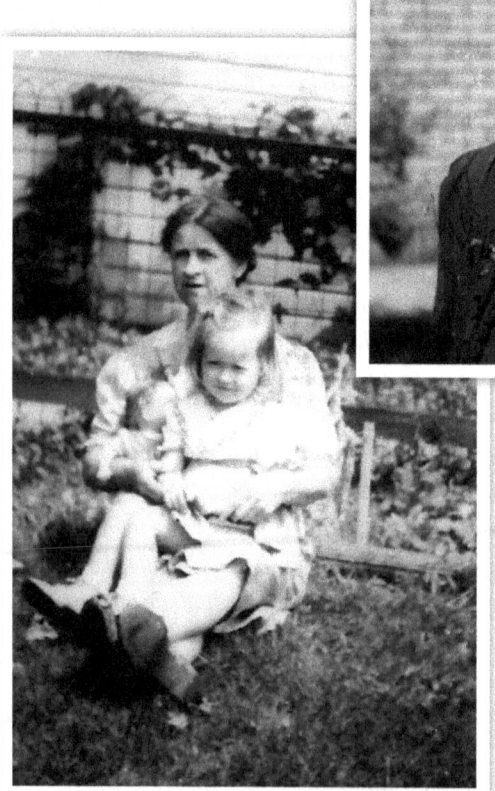

Grandma

Me and Grandma

CHAPTER 5
PET Scan
December 11, 2017

"We thought this was an infection because of how fast it came up. Cancers don't usually grow that quickly. It was kind of shocking. It was comforting to find out from Dolly that it was likely to be curable. Being physicians helped us deal with it." – Bob, son

Five days later, I was back at Rush for a PET scan.

The evening after my diagnosis was confirmed, I hadn't dissolved into tears. Occasionally my eyes would burn, but no actual tears, moaning, or other signs of grief overcame me. I still felt detached, as if this was happening to someone else. Not me!

Chris and I didn't talk about it much either. We agreed that I had to go through the motions, get the PET scan, talk to doctors some more. For a few days we went about our lives: shopped, cooked, did chores, worked on our computers, and sat in front of the television after dinner. My mind would drift to my concerns, and I'm sure Chris didn't concentrate so well either. He would have sensed my fears and had fears of his own. We both knew how we felt—words would have been superfluous.

But despite my continued doubts and inability to accept the reality of having cancer, I was now feeling anxious. A worrier all my adult life, my mind kept turning toward what the worst case might be. I felt jittery and lost my appetite. The day of the PET scan was no exception.

After I changed into a hospital gown in the radiology suite, a technician, a tall, intelligent-looking man with a warm demeanor, knocked, then came into the changing room and introduced himself. Nervously, I promptly forgot his name. I sat in a chair as he explained the test clearly and kindly.

"First, we'll give you an injection of glucose. Glucose is absorbed by cancer cells and makes them show up on the scan," he said. "Then we'll wait a bit to optimize the absorption before we put you through the scanner. That part is like having a CT scan. You lie still—it's important to be very still—and the machine will pass over you and take scans. It's going to scan you all the way from the tip of your head to your mid-thigh. Then the magic happens. Computers will match in 3-D any cancerous tissue that shows up on the scans to the findings on your CT. This will pinpoint for your doctors the exact location of each and every area they will have to treat, and areas they can avoid radiating."

The wonders of medical technology were impressive; however, it wasn't the procedure that frightened me, but the potential outcome.

The technician was asking, "You've had scans before. Does being in the scanner bother you?"

"I'm not nervous about the test itself. But I clear my throat and cough a lot. I hope I don't move too much and mess up the scan." I never had claustrophobia like some patients did during scans, but concentrating on staying immobile made me all the more squirmy.

"You'll be fine," he said. "Let's get started then."

After the PET scan, Chris and I walked across the street to Dr. Earvolino's office. She had read Dr. Thomas's notes and had the results of the PET scan by the time she saw us. The scan confirmed and defined a number of cancerous lymph nodes invading muscles on both sides of my neck. The lesion Dr. Thomas saw at the base of my tongue was identified as the primary lesion, the place where the cancer had started. There was no other cancer found anywhere else in my body.

This result was, of course, good. Not as good as, "It's all a mistake," but at least I could still be treatable.

Dr. Earvolino examined me, noting a dramatic decrease in the size of the lump under my right jaw, but still some unusual firmness where it had been. She also felt a small firm lump on the left side of my neck.

"How's your appetite?" she asked.

"Not too good. I can't eat when I'm nervous." I made a wry face. "I'm an incurable worrier."

I didn't want to take any medication for anxiety, but she talked me into a prescription for a low dose of lorazepam to have on hand if I needed it.

"Anxiety is natural, but we can't let it affect your appetite. You'll need energy to get through therapy, which is hard on your body. Don't refuse medications that can make your life easier. Take them only if you have to if you like, but there's no reason for you not to use them." She squeezed my hand.

My blood pressure was normal that day, but I told her I was concerned that cancer therapy would send my longstanding hypertension out of control. She explained that from now on my medical oncologist, who would be seeing me every week, would be managing my blood pressure and would make any medication changes that were needed.

I didn't like that plan. She had been my medical doctor for years. I wanted her! The thought made me feel lost.

"The nurses will be watching you closely. You'll be in constant touch with them. Don't try to guess ahead—they'll know what to do. It's best if I don't get in their way and complicate matters. Of course, if you feel you have to see me, please give me a call. Otherwise, I'll see you in six months, after you've recovered."

She patted my arm. "You're going to come through this."

I called Bob right away.

"It's the first bit of good news," I said. "At least the only cancer I have is what we already know about. My neck is back to normal, I have no symptoms at all, and I feel great. I still can't believe there's anything wrong with me."

"The scan *is* good news, Mom," he said, "but don't kid yourself. There are excellent results treating this kind of cancer, but you *do* have cancer."

Even though the idea of cancer scared me to death, if indeed I *did* have cancer, I told myself things could be worse. I wasn't going to risk my life based on my doubts. I had every confidence in my doctors and the medical center, especially after working there for so long and seeing first-hand their excellence. Not only were the surroundings familiar, but I believed there couldn't be a better place to treat my cancer. I would follow their advice, whatever that turned out to be. And I had two doctors in the family to hold my hand and help me make decisions—one of them an oncologist.

It was a matter of where to place my trust. All my life I had depended on myself to gather information and make decisions. Now I was learning that, in this crisis at least, others were better able to advise me. I trusted my husband, family, doctors, and the medical center. But did I trust them enough to take their advice over my own thoughts?

"I can't really take it all in yet, Bob. But I *am* scared. Of course—who wouldn't be? Thank God for you and Dolly! Have you warned her what a pest I can be when I'm stressed? I don't think she's seen that side of me."

"That should be the last of your worries, Mom. We'll get you through this."

It occurred to me then that if all this *was* true, regardless of how the lymph node got infected—by a dental condition or in some other way—we knew now that the cancer had already been present before I noticed the infection. Were it not for the coincidental infection, we wouldn't have discovered the cancer, and it would likely have continued to spread undetected and be well along by the time it was found. The infection may actually have saved my life.

God does, I thought, work in mysterious ways.

CHAPTER 6
Life Before Cancer: Child to Teen, 1948-1953

I can't remember a time when I wasn't an avid reader. My mother said I was reading by the age of two. What I think was true was that I was memorizing what she read to me and repeating words I remembered back to her with the pages open.

Whether or not I was actually reading that young, I credit my mother with inspiring my lifelong reading habit. She read to me every bedtime. My Aunt Isabel, who still lived in the flat downstairs with Grandma, bought me a new Little Golden Book every payday.

Before school age I was already familiar with our public library. We only went there in the summer months, when children were allowed to take out up to twenty books on "vacation loan" and keep them for three weeks.

My mother, my Aunt Isabel, and I walked to the library from our home near 55th and Christiana to the library at 62nd and Kedzie, over a mile one way. Yes, we walked in those days of one-car families, and kids walked too. We didn't need a First Lady to tell us we had to get plenty of exercise.

I would pick out my full quota of twenty books and read them in the backyard under the big old poplar tree as soon as we returned home. I usually finished all the books in a day or two.

"Mommy, is today library day?" I'd ask.

"No, we just went to the library yesterday."

"But…I read all my books, Mommy. Is tomorrow library day?"

"No, it's not. Read them again."

I usually wore her down before three weeks passed.

On vacations, while other children were playing, I would seek a quiet spot in a bedroom or curl up on a sofa or under a tree with a book.

My parents bought their first home—and, as it turned out, their only home—in 1953 and we moved to a modest frame ranch house in Oak Lawn, a popular middle-class suburb southwest of Chicago. I was eleven and my brother, Mike, was three.

I don't remember that Mike was as fond of reading as I was. He seemed more interested in playing outside and setting booby traps in the house. His favorite "inventions," as he called them, were arrangements of entangling ropes to walk into or things that would fall on us when we opened a door. My father never seemed to fall into his traps, but my mother and I did. He was pretty sneaky for a little kid—and, truth be told, pretty creative. An indication of the engineer he was to become?

With an eight-year difference between us, at a time when I was entering my teens and the independence that brings, Mike was pretty much relegated to the "annoying kid brother." In my mind, his booby traps served to reinforce that opinion. Yet I have clear memories of the coonskin cap and cowboy boots he wore not for dress-up but daily, and of getting down on all fours and allowing him to sit on my back for a "horsey-back ride," or holding him by one leg and one arm to spin him in circles, playing "helicopter." I also remember those poignant moments when he rushed into the house bursting to tell my mother or father something exciting. They didn't always want to interrupt what they were doing to listen to his prattle. I couldn't stand to see the hurt on Mike's little face, so I would call him over to tell me instead.

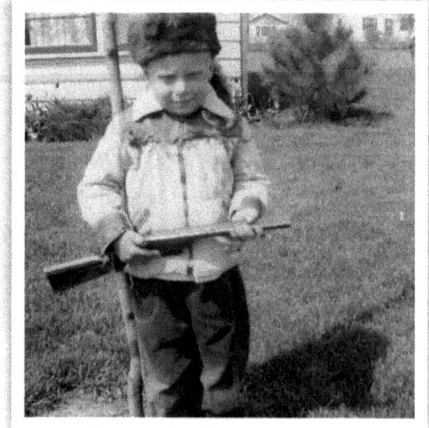

Mike wearing his coonskin cap.

CHAPTER 7
Consultation and Decision
Thursday, December 21, 2017

"Your mind raced at first, but as you learned more about your options, it seemed to ease your mind." – John, son

"I know today's treatments are very effective and patients do very well. No reason to panic or think the worst." - Dolly, daughter-in-law

I had an appointment to meet my care team mid-morning on Thursday, December 21: a medical oncologist, a radiation oncologist, and my ENT surgeon. I was told to expect to be there at least two hours. I could bring family members with me.

Christmas was only four days away. I didn't feel much like celebrating. The long holiday, however, made it possible for Bob and Dolly to clear their schedule and drive from their home in Fort Wayne to accompany Chris and me to the oncology consultation. Company in the house through the holiday would help me avoid thinking about my troubles, too.

The morning of the appointment, I lay in bed, peeking now and then at the morning sky through the upper part of our bedroom window, but mostly with my eyes shut and a queasy stomach, pretending to be asleep. Chris wasn't fooled. He curled his body around mine, spooning, his cheek against my hair.

"Are you ready for today?" he asked. His voice was almost a whisper. I knew he intended to be encouraging, but I recognized anxiety in his voice.

"I still can't believe this is happening—how can I be ready?" Not upset. Just stating a fact. I felt his warm breath ruffle my hair.

I could hear Bob and Dolly getting dressed in the spare bedroom. Mia would stay at our house with her nanny, Jenny, while we went to the hospital. Despite the fact that we were all heading out to plan my treatment, I clung to my hope that the diagnosis was all a big mistake. That's what the doctors would say today—we're so sorry, it's all a mistake, you don't have cancer after all.

I pushed my body more firmly against Chris. "I'm resigned, I guess. I have to go through this. My biggest fear is chemo. You know I get sick to my stomach for every little thing, and I hate that feeling. I'm a little nauseous *now*. Must be nerves. I might be vomiting for months. It's going to be hard…" My voice broke. "Really hard."

As long as I could remember I had a sensitive stomach. I vomited for the slightest thing: if I ate anything unusual, or a bit too much; if I exerted myself more than I was accustomed to; if I was anxious about something, even something I looked forward to. I remembered starting a vacation trip or a job interview with a cup beside me in case I couldn't keep my food down. On one occasion I was so excited to be joining friends at a restaurant that I spent the meal lying in the back seat of my car trying to keep from heaving instead of in the restaurant with everyone else. After such events I could count on waking up at two during the night to purge myself, spells that went on for a couple of hours and left me weak and trembling.

What I had to look forward to now was not only my customary lifelong dread of nausea and vomiting, but a disease and treatment that would almost certainly increase that specific misery.

Why now? Why does this have to happen right now, when my life is finally my own and going so well? When have I done enough to be able to enjoy "my time"?

Dealing with that fear, I had refused to talk about, or even think about, whether or not I would survive. Would two-year-old Mia, who I heard giggling in the next room, remember her grandmother a year from now?

Stop! Just stop! Get up and get moving! You're not doing yourself any good!

Later that morning, a medical assistant called us into an examining room in Rush's oncology department. When I worked at Rush, the oncology doctors' offices were in the Professional Building across the hall from my old office. The patient examination rooms were on the same floor, but at the other end of the building. I saw the doctors and patients every day, in the halls, in the restrooms. My familiarity with the surroundings was somewhat reassuring. The memory of some patients that wore wigs, were in wheelchairs, or looked emaciated was less assuring.

I was much more comfortable and confident at Rush than I would have been if I were seen elsewhere. Now that I had a serious disease, I was never more grateful for my former association with this medical institution.

I had dressed carefully. I wanted my new providers to think of me as professional, intelligent, and cooperative. I selected tan pants, a tan and black print knit top from Chico's, covered by a warm black fleece sleeveless vest. Black leather dress Oxfords completed the look. The outfit gave the impression I wanted, would keep me warm in Chicago winter, and allow me to pull up a sleeve or remove clothes easily for exams.

In my mind I had envisioned all of us sitting around a conference table in a large room full of doctors. Instead, we were led to a typical examination room, with a wall of windows that overlooked the walls of another building, an exam table, a desk with a computer and stool, and a side chair. I sat on the end of the exam table and Chris took the chair, while the assistant squeezed two more chairs into the crowded space for Bob and Dolly.

While driving the ninety minutes it took to go from Lemont to the medical center during rush hour on the Stevenson Expressway, we made small talk. Now, we sat in silence, nervously avoiding each other's eyes. I felt like I should be saying something, but I didn't.

After about ten minutes, a short, slender, dark-skinned man wearing black pants, a white shirt, and a maroon tie came into the room, held his hand out to me, and introduced himself as Dr. Layan.

"I'm your radiation oncologist," he said. "I specialize in head and neck cancer, and I'm here to explain what we propose as the best treatment for you."

He seemed very young to me, and I wondered for a moment if he was a fellow or a resident. I need not have worried, as his words, professional manner, and brilliance were soon evident.

He seated himself on the computer stool and got right to the point. "We talked about your case at tumor board," he said. He spoke slowly and softly. "Dr. Thomas was part of that conversation. He said he had discussed a surgical option with you, called a radical neck dissection. It's a seven-hour surgery to remove the tumor as well as the lymph nodes in your neck."

"He said he hoped we'd be able to avoid that," I said. I had purposely not looked up descriptions of facial disfigurement. I didn't really want to consider the possibility. But now an image of an elderly woman missing part of her lower jaw formed in my mind.

"Yes, and that's what we all agreed. We're recommending a research study for you—a trial. We feel your cancer will respond to a more conservative treatment of radiation and chemotherapy alone. You would need radiation and chemotherapy even if you had the surgery, but we feel we'll get a good result without the surgery."

He watched me for a few moments. When I said nothing, he continued.

"The standard treatment is for radiation of a large area of your head, neck, and upper chest to destroy the tumor in your tongue as well as any existing cancer in your head and neck. This is done along with chemotherapy in the event that microscopic cancer that was not seen on your studies has spread to other areas of your body. Even if you had the surgery, as I said, you would still have to have a similar therapy."

He waited while an "L" train rumbled by loudly outside the windows on the tracks between the buildings.

"But you said you're suggesting a trial. That means not having the surgery?"

"Yes. The trial is based on good evidence that less radiation and an alternate drug is effective for the particular kind of cancer you have."

He leaned toward me, placing his elbows on his knees and keeping eye contact. "The head and neck are full of vital structures. Tailoring radiation to avoid injury to these structures while destroying the cancer is not an easy task. But we can do this using details from your PET scan and computer mapping. We can direct your radiation dose using the lowest exposure, and more selectively to the smallest area possible, targeting only the areas we know are cancerous plus the most likely areas for spread. This does not mean you will have *no* side effects, but the side effects will be reduced."

I was hesitant. I didn't want side effects and disfiguring surgery, of course. And—awful thought—pain and nausea. But if I did anything, I wanted the best chance for cure. I wasn't sure he understood my fears.

"If I go with the trial, is it enough? …uh…what happens if I have the radiation and chemo and you don't get it all, and I still have cancer?"

His gaze met mine. "Then you have the surgery."

"Not more radiation and chemo?"

"No. We do this one time."

There was silence in the room while I looked at the floor and let that sink in. One chance his recommendation would work. A good chance, he said. Or radical surgery.

"What are the risks of the trial?"

"There's always a risk—medicine is not an exact science. And there are still side effects, but they're less. However, we feel this is the best option for you, that it's safe, and that you'll have a good result. You are, in fact, an ideal candidate for the study."

"But this is my decision? I can have the surgery—if that's what I want. Or the standard treatment?"

"Yes, you decide."

I paused again. "If I was your mother, what would you be telling her to do?"

Without hesitation, he said, "I'd tell her to go for the trial."

I swallowed hard. I clasped my hands together in my lap to stop them from shaking, and looked away from the doctor to Chris, Bob, and Dolly.

"What do you think?" My voice sounded to my ears as if it came from a distance over the pounding of my heart.

Dolly spoke up. "You've asked all the right questions, Pat. I'm familiar with this study and I think it's the right thing to do. For squamous cell cancer, which you have, the results are very good. We can cure this kind of cancer now. You're lucky to have this option."

I turned and looked at Bob. "You're in good hands, Mom. Let the experts do what they do."

Finally, I looked at Chris. After a long moment, he nodded. Tears burned in my eyes but didn't fall. I turned to Dr. Layan and nodded too.

"Good," he said. "Let me examine you."

He looked in my mouth and probed my neck gently but thoroughly.

"My swelling is almost gone now, but it was the size of a plum before Dr. Thomas drained it," I said.

While Dr. Layan examined me, he told me more about the treatment. Some of it didn't sink in, and I knew I wouldn't remember everything, but I trusted that Dolly and Bob would do that. I was glad he kept talking, though, because his voice was calming.

"We'll give you a binder today to take home. It explains everything. You'll come in five days a week for eight weeks. Pretty soon the treatment will affect your taste buds and your salivary glands. Your mouth will be dry, and you won't want to eat all the foods you normally eat. Expect your appetite to be poor, and you'll lose weight, so we'll have a dietitian follow you. Toward the end of radiation, the skin on your neck will burn, but aside from that you shouldn't have too much discomfort. The burning will start slowly and increase over the course of radiation and will continue to get worse after treatment for a while. That's the effect of radiation, but you will also be having chemotherapy at the same time, which has its own side effects."

"Will I be nauseous? I'm really scared of that."

"We don't expect that from radiation, but perhaps from chemotherapy. Dr. Fidler, your medical oncologist, will explain that."

He reached into his shirt pocket and pulled out a card, which he handed to me. "My email and cell phone number. Contact me any time you have questions, problems, or just want to talk. You'll hear from our office with a schedule of your appointment dates and times. We'll start in about three weeks. I'll see you then. Wait here now for Dr. Fidler. She'll be in shortly."

As soon as Dr. Layan left the room, Chris got up and put his arms around me.

Bob said, "You made the right decision, Mom."

Dolly nodded. "I liked him."

Chris still had one arm around me when Dr. Fidler entered the room. She shook his hand, then mine, and nodded to Bob and Dolly before seating herself behind the computer.

Dr. Mary Jo Fidler was a short, thirty-something woman with curly light-brown hair, kind light-blue eyes, a pleasant smile, and a quiet, professional demeanor. She was rather plump, and almost looked as if she was pregnant. I wondered if she *was* pregnant. After Dr. Thomas told us her name, we looked up her credentials and found that she had published extensively and was a leading expert in the field of oncology. To me, she looked like any other young mother, perhaps a neighbor.

After we all identified ourselves, she asked, ""How did you like Dr. Layan?"

I exchanged glances with my family. "We thought he was great," I said, smiling.

"Well, he explained the radiation part to you. I'm a medical oncologist, like your daughter-in-law." She nodded at Dolly. "Radiation alone won't stop your cancer, because it has already spread. Surgery won't stop it either, if we were recommending that. You will need chemotherapy, and that will be done at the same time as radiation."

She spoke slowly and softly, like Dr. Layan had. "The standard treatment is a drug called Cisplatin. But Cisplatin has a lot of side effects, one of the most troublesome being vomiting. Some people can't tolerate it and have to be taken off treatment early."

"Yes," I interrupted. "I'm especially afraid of that. I get nauseous for the smallest thing."

"We can give you medication to help with the nausea, but the trial we've recommended doesn't include Cisplatin. You'll be getting a drug called Cetuximab. It's not actually a chemotherapy agent, but a monoclonal antibody that's effective for your particular cancer. Cetuximab has its own side effects, but less than you would have with Cisplatin. Some people don't have nausea at all."

Dolly said, "Cetuximab is a good choice, Pat. It'll be much easier on you than Cisplatin, and it's very effective."

I wasn't convinced. I wanted the *best* treatment, not the easiest. I wanted this cancer *gone*! "But you said Cisplatin is the usual drug. Is it more effective than Cetuximab? Is Cetuximab experimental?"

Dr. Fidler shook her head. "No to both questions. The FDA approved Cetuximab for treatment of head and neck cancers in 2006. It works in a different way than Cisplatin. Cisplatin kills cancer cells directly, but it can't distinguish between cancer cells and healthy cells, which is why there are so many side effects. Cetuximab works by recognizing and attaching to cancer cells specifically and working along with the body's immune system to attack only abnormal cells."

Dolly was nodding. "It's a good drug. Especially for colon cancer and squamous cell cancers of the head and neck, which is what you have." She and Dr. Fidler exchanged glances.

"So, Cisplatin wouldn't increase my chances for a cure?"

"You might call it overkill," Bob said. He was probably trying to lighten things up. I shot him a dirty look, but I didn't mean it. No one laughed.

Dr. Fidler stood up and examined me, looking in my mouth and feeling my neck, the same as Dr. Layan had done. Her touch was gentle and reassuring, as his had been. She listened to my heart and lungs, asked me to lie down, and felt my abdomen. I remembered she would be acting as my medical doctor as well as my oncologist during therapy, as Dr. Earvolino had mentioned.

Sitting back on her stool, she explained, "We'll start chemotherapy the same time you start radiation, but chemo is once a week, while radiation is five days. The first dose will be what we call a 'loading dose.' We give a stronger dose to give you a boost at the beginning. There will be a total of eight doses, or eight weeks. Our secretaries will make the appointments and get in touch with you. After each dose, someone will have to drive you home." She looked at Chris.

"Of course," he said. "I'll be with her for all her appointments. Is it possible to avoid rush hour? We come about thirty miles."

"Late morning, then, or early afternoon. We'll coordinate with radiation and let you know."

Dr. Fidler stood up, put her hand on my arm, and squeezed gently. "Good," she said, looking directly in my eyes. "We're going to take good care of you. Now wait here and someone will be in to bring you the papers you need to sign to agree to enter the study. She'll also give you materials to take home and read."

The clinical coordinator for the research study was Mandy, a tall, large-boned woman in her early thirties who managed to be both businesslike and warm. She went over the information and consent forms, and I signed the papers, which were extensive but well organized. We walked out with a binder and folders explaining all that we had agreed to and what to expect over the course of treatment. I'd be busy studying the materials much of the time left before treatment began.

On the way out, I stopped at a desk where I was introduced to Julie. She gave me a card and told me she would be making all my appointments, and I was to call her if I had any questions or needed to reach Dr. Fidler.

Chris, Bob, and Dolly made encouraging comments on the drive home and then tried to distract me with other topics. Eventually I dropped my head back, closed my eyes, and withdrew into my own thoughts, tormented by doubt.

Had I made the right choice? I wasn't confident. Why was I going to be making myself sick when I didn't feel sick? Why fix something that didn't feel broken? Especially if fixing it meant making myself miserable for months. Who knew how long it would be before I was back to normal?

I had always been able to see an issue from all sides, and that was usually thought to be a good thing. I viewed this ability as a curse rather than a blessing. Understanding all options makes it much harder to make decisions. It limits the things one can be passionate about, because you can see the benefits of each choice, as well as the negatives, and every choice seems equal.

Who knew if the choice I made would work? Since it seemed I really had cancer, should I be taking the easy route? Maybe I should take the standard route, have the surgery, the extensive radiation, the established drug. But I trusted the doctors at Rush. The medical people in my own family thought this was the best thing to do, and all these people knew a whole lot more than I did. Were it not for that, I probably would have taken the harder course, but according to what they all said, there was no good reason to do that.

It didn't occur to me yet that the treatment itself might leave me impaired in some permanent way that could affect my life and my ability to do things that were important to me, such as singing. At that time, I thought more about survival and what the treatment would be like.

I decided I would tough it out despite my doubts and do the best I could to follow what I was told. Any other attitude was likely to make my journey worse.

My treatment would start with the new year, on January 2.

CHAPTER 8
Life Before Cancer:
New Friends and Reading, 1953-1960

*I*n my new neighborhood, I felt like I didn't belong at first because I was the "new kid." My classmates didn't like me much because I frequently waved my hand to correct a student that had given a wrong answer in class. I had transferred from a Catholic school where the nuns had taught us to correct every answer that wasn't exactly right. I thought that was what I was supposed to do, and I was anxious to please. I didn't please, of course, but angered the other kids. Even my own cousin, who was in my class.

"What's wrong with her?" some boy whose name I don't remember complained to my cousin within my hearing. "Miami was the right answer, but she has to stick up her hand and say it was Miami, Florida. Everyone knows Miami is in Florida, and we were talking about Florida!"

"It's not my fault she's my cousin. I don't know why she does that!" My cousin was clearly embarrassed by me.

I quickly learned that what the nuns taught me in that regard was not transferable to my new school. I've been overly sensitive about correcting anyone ever since.

I noticed another girl who didn't quite belong, but for different reasons. Carolyn had skipped a grade because she was ahead of other fifth-grade students and joined my sixth-grade class. I'd seen her riding her bicycle alone in a noticeably purposeful way. Her long dark hair streamed behind her, halfway down her back. She probably thought she was better than the other kids, I supposed. I didn't realize at the time I was making the same impression. As temporary sixth-grade misfits, Carolyn and I soon became friends. It turned out we had many of the same interests, especially in horses, libraries, and books.

That summer following sixth grade Carolyn and I would ride our bicycles to the Oak Lawn Library at least once a week, more often if we ran out of books. We rode Schwinn bikes with fat tires, a rear "seat" for passengers, and a basket hanging from the handlebars.

The library was in an old house that dated back to Civil War days, two small dark rooms, crowded with shelves, the only furniture a desk where the single librarian used a rubber stamp to check out the books we selected. There was no place to sit except on the floor, and sometimes we did that. The wooden floors creaked and were so badly slanted that anything you dropped would roll out of sight. There was a narrow creek at the edge of the property, where no one ever went. Carolyn and I would lie on the little bridge that crossed the stream to read the books we'd just checked out. When it got late, we'd get our bikes, fill our baskets with stacks of books, and wobble home.

Carolyn and I were both obsessed with horses at the time, a passion that didn't interest our other friends. Our favorite books were horse stories, especially those written by Walter Farley and Marguerite Henry, the Westerns and dog stories of Thomas C. Hinkle, and more.

Thomas Hinkle wrote wonderful books about the American West, the herds of wild horses and cattle dogs that roamed there, and the men who were the horses' enemies and became their friends. Hinkle grew up on the plains of Kansas in the late 1800s when covered wagons still crossed the plains. Many of his books were based on true stories. His books are lost to today's readers—probably because they seem pretty lame compared to graphic novels and vampires—but we loved them. Once we exhausted the Hinkle books the library owned, we anxiously awaited new volumes to appear on the shelves, but they never did. We didn't know at the time that he had died ten years before we discovered his books.

We weren't called young adults then—we were teen readers. The point is, reading was a big part of our lives and inspired a lifelong friendship.

As more friends came into my circle, one of my favorite activities was to *play school, where I was "teacher" and urged all my "class" to read. Not just during playtime, but even in bed at night I dreamed up "school" activities. I fell into the role of teacher naturally and found that I flourished when I became the person in charge. Which was probably why later I fell into an administrative career, that is in many ways similar to teaching with additional responsibilities.*

Others might have called me bossy, and I can't argue with that.

My reading preferences underwent an abrupt change when I was about thirteen. One summer day, out of boredom, I wandered through our attic and found an entire box of paperback Perry Mason mysteries. Curious, I asked my mother if I could read them. She thought I was a bit young, but gave in. I read every one of them that summer, and mysteries became my new favorite genre.

I'm not quite sure why I liked mysteries so much. Perhaps I liked the idea that someone, some person with only intelligence as a tool, noticed things others overlooked and put together little clues to solve a seemingly impossible puzzle in real life. An ordinary sort of skill that most anyone could develop if they tried hard enough. At the end the sleuth would do something no one else had been able to do, and there was satisfaction in that. The fact that someone else was humbled or punished as a result of his efforts was satisfying too.

I gravitated toward fiction, not at first realizing why. Later I realized that I also favored longform fiction to short stories. I wanted to be with my characters over a long period of time and feel a part of their lives in a way that was not as satisfying in a short story. Short stories made me feel rushed. I can relax with a novel, and that's why I read.

No matter where I lived or what I did throughout my life, there have always been libraries, filled with adventures about whatever interested me at the time. Sometimes they were little two-room old buildings, other times mid-sized suburban, large city, or university libraries. I sought them out wherever I lived. Regardless of size and facilities, all libraries have had something to endear them to me. They all provide refuge from the stresses of life.

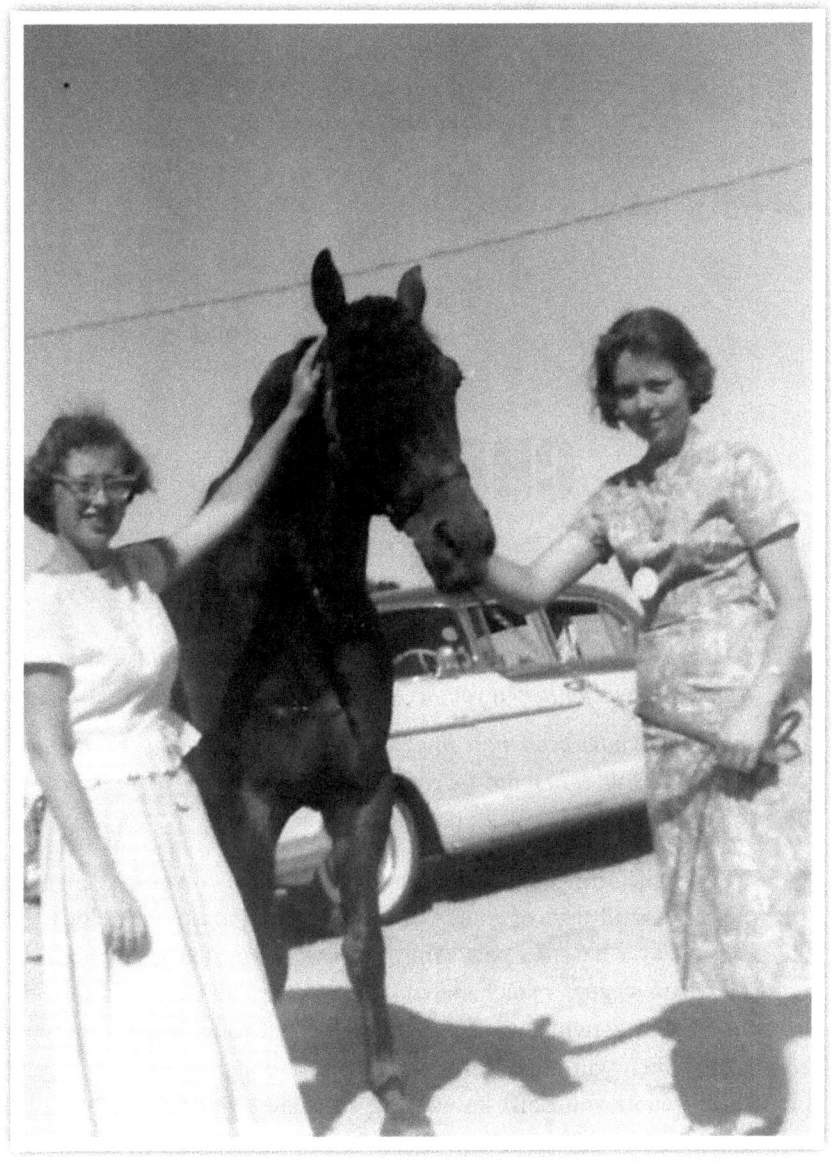

Me and Carolyn, the "horse" years.

CHAPTER 9

Christmas
December 22, 2017 through December 25, 2017

"I know you are a strong woman and hoped that strength wouldn't keep you from asking us for help if you needed it." - Clare, daughter-in-law

"I wish we could have been more involved. Mia was still in diapers and had to be fed at certain times. But we got to spend the holidays all together." – Dolly, daughter-in-law

Here's the thing about cancer—it's insidious. If you've caught it early—and that, of course, is the best thing to do—you don't feel sick, you have no pain. You feel fine. If you felt lousy, you'd be motivated to do whatever you had to do to get better. But when you feel fine, first you have to convince yourself something is wrong, because nothing feels wrong. Then you must learn to trust mind-boggling technology and a bunch of people you don't know. And even after you do that, you still ask yourself why you're about to get started—willingly—on something that's probably going to make you feel worse than you ever have in your life.

Tell me again—why the hell am I doing this?

I had been surprised to learn that I had to wait almost two weeks to begin chemotherapy and radiation, but the delay was necessary for surgery scheduling and planning details. I had expected to get started right away.

Wouldn't the disease progress while I waited? My doctors assured me that treatment was really happening rapidly, and two weeks would not affect the outcome in any way, but I was still disappointed. Now that I'd agreed, I wanted to get started and get it over with. Nor did I want to start second-guessing my decision.

The delay turned out to be useful. Once I began cancer therapy, most likely my activities would be limited, and I had a lot of matters to settle beforehand. Although my therapy would end early in March, recovery would take another three months, or longer, my doctors said. So, I was looking at about six months away from normal activity. Also, I needed to fit in some medical appointments before treatment began.

Two days after the consultation, Bob accompanied me when I returned to my dentist. If I needed any extractions, root canals, or major dental work it should be done first, so as not to interrupt treatment. Radiation would affect my salivary glands, causing dry mouth. Saliva helps prevent tooth decay, so I would be prone to tooth disease, and radiation could cause bone loss, which could affect my jaw. I'd need fluoride treatments, probably lifelong. If I needed dental work, it could delay the beginning of treatment for my cancer.

My cancer came from my tongue, but I didn't realize initially that getting rid of cancer could involve so many other medical and dental complications. I was finding out there was a *lot* involved.

My dentist seemed a little relieved that my problem was not a dental issue after all.

"I'm not a strong believer in fluoride treatments," he said. "But certainly, if your doctors think they'll be helpful I'm happy to give them to you."

He did a thorough oral examination and assured me that my teeth looked sound and my mouth healthy. He prepared a letter to clear me for the planned treatment and gave me a bottle of prescription-strength fluoride rinse, told me to brush and floss more frequently than usual, use the softest toothbrush I could find and a Waterpik, and replace mouthwash with Biotene for dry mouth.

He wished me well. "You're fortunate to have found this so early," he said as he walked with me to the front of his office. I introduced him to Bob and they shook hands. My dentist turned back to me. "I'm sure you'll do well. Please call me, or have your doctors call me, if there's anything I can do."

My family would be staying with us until the morning after Christmas. Meanwhile, with extra people in the house, I kept busy and distracted reading book after book to Mia, a bright and sweet child, who was as passionate about reading as I had been at her age. We all tried to avoid talking about my cancer, and I ran out of questions for Bob and Dolly, who were in and out of the house a lot—shopping, wrapping, and visiting.

In bed at night, however, I was still tortured by doubt. *What am I more afraid of—having cancer or the treatment of my cancer? Since I feel so well, I guess that's why I'm not getting the full impact of having cancer. My head knows I could die from this, but the thought seems so remote. This can't really be happening to me!*

Thank God for my good doctors, my supportive family, my good friends. It's a relief to have doctors I'm familiar with, a place I'm familiar with—a place I have so much confidence in. Thank God I had the good fortune to work for so many years at one of the best medical centers in the world.

But I still have to go through this. Me—I'm a cancer patient. I'm in good hands, but I don't really know what that's going to be like. What's going to happen to me?

I turned onto my back. A picture came to my mind from more than thirty years ago: the pained, defeated expression on the face of a breast cancer patient we were treating in our office. As I entered notes in her chart, she sat at the end of the exam table, a thin, average-height woman with uncombed lanky dark hair, propped against the table's upright back. She held a partly filled emesis basin, her head hanging onto her chest, her husband helping to steady her. She looked exceedingly weak, her eyes unfocused, her skin pale and yellowish. When she left the office, her husband and a nurse had to almost carry her out to her car. I never saw her again, but I learned that her chemotherapy had to be discontinued because she couldn't tolerate her vomiting. She died not long afterward.

Would what happened to her happen to me? That incident happened more than twenty years ago. Surely there had been advances in medical science since then. The memory made me realize that my fear of nausea and vomiting wasn't just because I didn't like to get sick. Knowing how susceptible I was, there was a risk vomiting could be severe enough that I wouldn't be able to finish cancer treatment, and I would die.

On Christmas Day, Bob drove all of us out to John and Clare's home in Sycamore, about an hour away. I usually cooked dinner for whoever could make it to our house for all the holidays, so it seemed a little strange to let someone else do the work. However, I hadn't done any holiday shopping, not for family dinners and not for Christmas gifts. My focus, ever since Thanksgiving, had been on medical care.

I was grateful that our whole family could be together for the day, but embarrassed that I didn't have a pile of gifts for everyone that year. A card and money didn't put delight in a two-year-old's eyes. However, my family pitched in and there were plenty of gifts from others to go around, and I doubt my omissions were even noticed.

In fact, the day turned out just about perfect. Not having the burden of preparing and entertaining, getting more exhausted as the day wore on, it was a pleasure to sit back and watch others do the work this time. I got to relax and enjoy my grandchildren.

John, like many engineers, was particular about his environment and his activities. He liked to be with people but preferred to go elsewhere rather than entertain. But when he did entertain, he took pains to do it right.

Clare, on the other hand, grew up in a large and somewhat chaotic Irish family, and was easy-going and tended toward being a people-pleaser. So, as I sat at his kitchen table watching Clare and Dolly prepare the meal, I was not surprised that John was doing much of the preparation. Chris, Bob, the three grandchildren, and Jenny, Mia's nanny, were in the adjacent great room, some watching television and others playing games.

"I'm not exactly an invalid—yet!" I said. "Can't I help?"

"We want to treat you," Clare said. "Just enjoy yourself. You've entertained us more times than we can count. Let us take a turn."

Clare was an artist, with a master's degree in fashion design and an eye for color and decoration. Dolly also crafted artistic projects in the scarce free time left to her after treating patients. Soon the two were chattering about their respective craft projects. John didn't mind being shut out, as he tended to be task-focused.

I drifted into the great room, where a Christmas tree sat in a corner between the fireplace and front windows. It was lovely. My daughters-in-law were much better at decorating than me. I was the collector, who took out the same old things I'd been using for years, things my mother had used, and a few new items picked up most likely at Dollar Tree.

Collin, my oldest grandchild, was now eighteen. He didn't seem to know what to talk to me about. We spent some time conversing about his plans for college since he would be starting soon. I sensed that he was concerned about what would happen to me, but although we could usually talk easily about day-to-day matters and general topics, personal feelings would be awkward for a teenager. Even adults don't know what to say to people who have cancer.

Everyone was busy except me. I grabbed Mia and picked up a tote bag full of books. "Let's go to the living room and read. Would you like that?"

I needn't have asked. Mia loved being read to more than any other activity.

After dinner we opened gifts. No one seemed to mind that they had only cards and money from Chris and me. Chris was generous but was not a good gift shopper. Well, he had suggestions and opinions, but he didn't know what children like. So, gift shopping was generally left to me.

Aidan, fourteen that Christmas, had decided that I would need some items to keep me comfortable during my radiation. He made me a neck pillow and another pillow filled with rice that I could warm in the microwave and wrap over painful areas. I was delighted with his thoughtfulness but didn't tell him that I wouldn't be putting something warm over the burns I expected to be the only pain I would be having.

"Can I take you for your surgery?" John asked.

"John, that's nice of you to offer, but won't you have to be back to work?"

"I can take off." It wasn't as easy as he was making it sound, I knew. He worked long hours at a nuclear power plant and was called on frequently to solve problems.

"Please. Chris will be with me. It's just a biopsy, a simple procedure, not a big deal."

If I expected a traumatic experience, I would have wanted him there. Bob too. But I expected only a minor procedure, not a traumatic experience.

"What about radiation and chemo? Don't you need us then? John and I can alternate taking days off," Clare said.

"Really, Chris will be with me for every appointment. We'll be fine."

"Maybe we can bring you some meals, then," John said, looking at Clare for confirmation.

"How about if I stop by with some Crock-Pot meals, so you don't have to cook," Clare said.

"Thanks, but it's silly for you to drive an hour and back on a workday when we can easily run out for fast food. It won't hurt our diet for a few months. Besides, I don't know what I'll be able to eat, and Chris isn't fussy. I plan to fill the refrigerator and pantry with things he likes anyway."

I could see they were sincere, but I also saw relief on their faces. It wasn't just words on my part. Yes, they did have their own lives that I didn't want to stress. Chris and I *would* be alone. But I wouldn't have to pretend to be brave to Chris. We could face what was to come together, but it meant more than I could say that my family was willing to be there and to help.

I was moved almost to tears. The most important thing to me was that they were all there with me when I needed them. I had such a loving, supportive family. Just what I would need to get me through what was soon to come—whether it was minor or terrible.

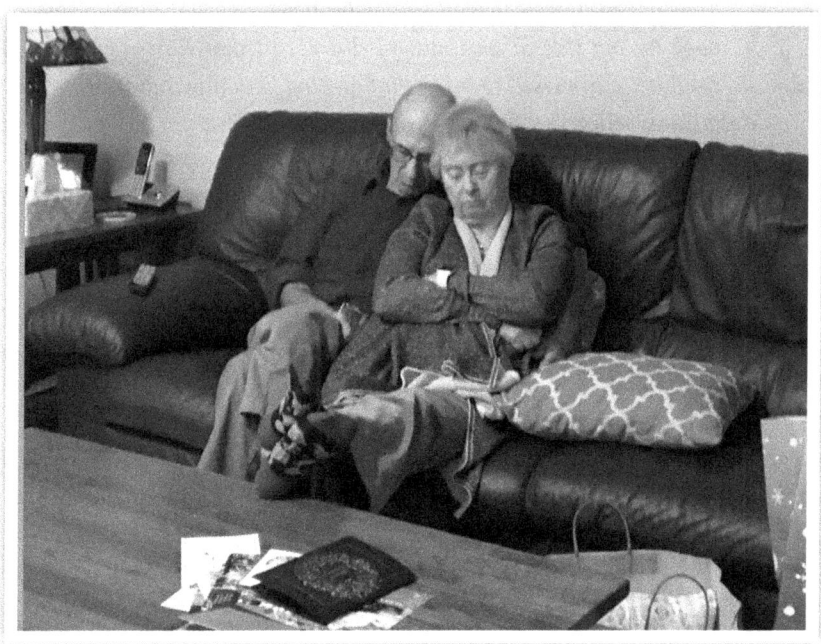

Chris and me, Christmas, 2017. Showing the strain.

CHAPTER 10
Life Before Cancer: College, Marriage, and Motherhood, 1960-1968

Although I continued to read avidly through high school and college—a book by my side at all times—I did not at that time have enough confidence in myself to think that writing fiction was ever something I could do. So in college I dithered between studying literature or biology and in my sophomore year decided on biology.

The college I attended, Saint Xavier, was at that time an all-girl liberal arts college. Although most of us expected to marry and become housewives, we valued the confidence and pride that came from a liberal education. In my junior year I met Frank. We shared a lot of laughs with friends and seemed to share interests and goals. By the time I graduated in 1965, we were engaged to marry that summer.

While completing my education, I concentrated on getting my biology degree, with little thought given to how I would use the degree once I had it. I minored in education, so I was qualified to teach if that interested me. After graduation, I discovered the truth: an undergraduate degree in biology was useless by itself. I either had to get additional skilled training or an advanced degree. This glitch in the career path didn't upset me much. Since I would be married that summer, I accepted a job as a seventh-grade teacher in a parochial school. I thought I'd have time to figure out my career after teaching for a year or two.

Unlike many young women, I never felt a strong attraction to babies or children. But I surprised myself when John was born in 1966. Oh my! Holding your own child! The feelings that came over me were indescribable. That boundless love. Like a combination of joy and tenderness, a wave that filled my chest and left no room for any other thought or emotion. Except perhaps for a bit of terror: I would be solely responsible for the life and wellbeing of this tiny man in my arms.

I discovered that I loved being a mother. And, of course, my son was beautiful, and no other child compared to him. So, when I got pregnant with Bob before John's first birthday, I was delighted to think I might have another child just like John. I imagine I'm not unlike other mothers who assumed their second child would be a carbon copy of the first. In my foolishness that's what I thought, and of course I was wrong. Bob, born in 1967, was nothing like John in any way. But I loved him just as much.

I remember writing a letter to a favorite teacher during those years of my sons' early childhood, trying to explain how my love for my children was equal but different. I ended by describing love as an intense relationship between two people, which could never be the same because the object of each relationship differed. But in every case the love could be just as strong.

Although many women would say that raising two sons, only sixteen months apart, was exhausting and confining, looking back I think that time may have been the years I felt most free. My responsibilities as a mother were the same as any other mother, but I had few other responsibilities—no job, no parents to care for. I ran my home as I pleased. When there was something I wanted to do, such as go to the library, I put the boys in a buggy and off we went. When my sons napped, I had the afternoon to myself, and more time after they went to bed in the evening.

I hadn't been much of a worrier in my early years, but being a mother soon changed that. If my boys were late waking, I'd immediately think the worst, imagining crib death. If I left an open jar of baby food in the refrigerator too long, I'd worry that I poisoned them. If they were out of my sight they were lost or doing something dangerous. Once learned, habitual worrying spread to all aspects of my life and took effort to control.

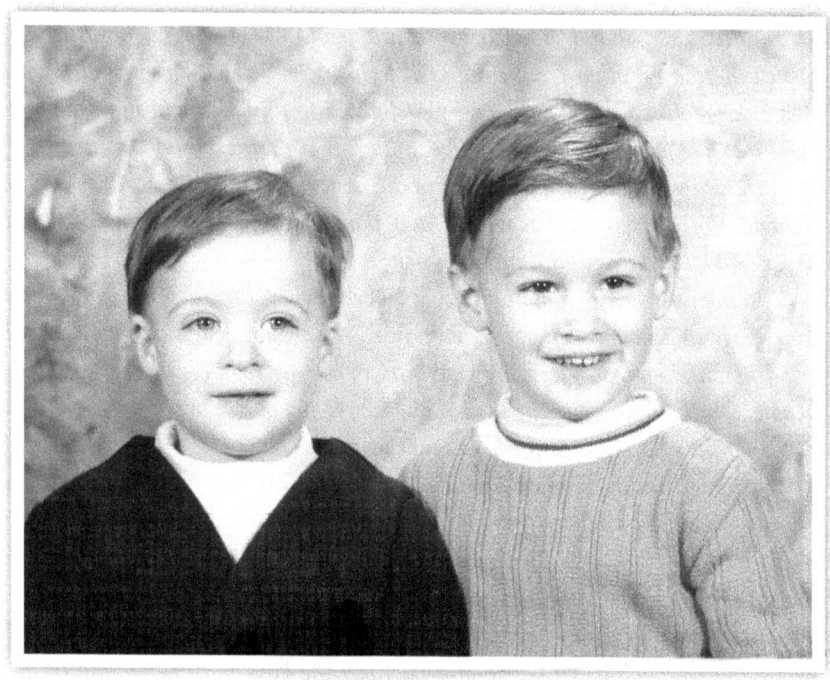

Bob (age 2) and John (age 3)

CHAPTER 11
After Christmas
December 26, 2017

"I wanted to be available and a sounding board, to be someone you could talk to...but I saw you getting what you needed on your own." - John, son

The next morning, Tuesday, December 26, Bob and Dolly returned to Fort Wayne. I wanted nothing more than to creep back into bed, recover my energy, and be alone to wrestle with my emotions, but I had yet another appointment that morning. Dr. Thomas wanted to see me again, this time for preoperative evaluation.

After arrival, Chris and I were taken to an exam room where an assistant drew some blood and took an electrocardiogram, tests the hospital required for surgical clearance. When Dr. Thomas arrived, he greeted me, not with his usual cheery, "What's happening?" but today he asked, "How are you doing?"

"Okay, so far," I said, with a crooked grin. "Not so sure how I'll be by Tuesday."

"Well, let's talk about this." I hadn't seen him in person since before the diagnosis was confirmed. He sat on a stool and looked in my eyes, his face appearing kind but serious.

"Let's review what we're doing," he went on. "That lump in your neck is almost completely gone, but before we drained it, we were probably looking at what we call a metastatic adenopathy from that lesion I saw at the base of your tongue. Before we can start treating you, we'll need to do an examination under anesthesia and a biopsy to be sure that tongue mass is the cause of all the cancer we found."

"Can't you do it with the scope?"

"We *will* be using a scope, but we need to look further and that would be too uncomfortable for you. Especially with the instruments we use. So, we do it under anesthetic. You wouldn't like me very much if we didn't." He grinned.

I nodded but frowned. I was weighing my decision for discomfort versus what I expected the risks and recovery from anesthetic would be like. General anesthesia scared me. I hated the thought of losing control while someone was cutting on my body. But maybe it wasn't so bad to be asleep and wake up knowing the surgery was over. Surely Dr. Thomas knew what was best.

"There are minor risks with a direct laryngoscopy and biopsy. It could be hard to control bleeding. Anesthesia complications like allergy, difficulty passing the tube, breathing problems, injury to your airway or teeth. After the surgery you can expect to have a sore throat, but it shouldn't be too bad nor last too long—the biopsy site and the anesthesia tube can leave you with some discomfort. There's also a slight risk of perforation during the procedure." He placed his hand over my wrist, his expression compassionate. "I do a lot of these procedures, and I can tell you these things almost never happen."

I wasn't very worried about complications because of my experience working with surgeons and told him so.

"I know complications are rare, and I trust you. I'm more worried about being sick after the procedure…and the outcome."

He smiled. "Thank you. We have options to make you comfortable. You're in good general health, and I feel confident you'll do well."

Even though I was hearing, "You'll do well," over and over, his words still gave me a sense of relief.

"So now, one other thing. Sometimes patients with your condition experience hearing difficulties as a result of treatment. So we'd like to have a baseline, to know what your hearing is like before we start. Our audiologist can test you today while you're here. When she's finished, come back to this room and I'll do another laryngoscopy in preparation for next week. Then you can go home."

I was a bit surprised, both to learn that my hearing was at risk and by how thorough the preparation was. But I was also reassured by the thoroughness. The detailed care reinforced the reasons I go to an academic medical center, where these options are readily available.

My audiogram was essentially normal, with only a little loss in the high frequencies and no change from a test I'd had four years ago. That was good. The laryngoscopy also went well. An assistant gave me a booklet called "What You Need to Know About Your Procedure" and a sheet that described the potential for hearing or balance loss due to toxicity from chemotherapy. I was almost sad when Dr. Thomas left the office because his presence had been so comforting.

Already appointments were taking over my life, and now I was left with seven days before I no longer decided my own schedule.

With Christmas past and Chris and I alone again, worry threatened to overwhelm me. I had to get my head on straight and sort out personal matters.

First, I read the patient education information I'd been given: the study prospectus, the multiple pamphlets and instruction guides. More questions, and more doubts, cropped up.

If my cancer or my treatment could affect my voice and my hearing, how was that going to affect my career as a writer? To promote sales of the books I had written, I scheduled frequent speaking engagements and book signings. I would have to cancel those during treatment, but would I recover well enough to return? Would I still be able to sing, or would I have to give up the chorus I enjoyed so much? I had finally reached a point in life where I had time available to enjoy these activities. I was just settling in and now everything had to come to an abrupt stop. I felt gypped.

My activities enriched my quality of life and pleasure, but what about more basic survival? What would I be able to eat? Would I be able to eat *at all*? Or would I need a feeding tube? It seemed that most patients with my cancer had to be fed by tube. My mother had had a feeding tube when she became unable to swallow. The tube kept her alive for years, but it wasn't very pleasant, and I had distinct memories of taking care of her at the time. Would the same thing happen to me? If so, would I be able to get off the tube after I recovered? Not all patients did.

Was I healthy enough to withstand chemotherapy and radiation? Would my blood pressure go out of control? What if the radiation caused so much swelling it cut off my airway and I couldn't breathe? Any of these things could happen.

My fears were beginning to get beyond my control. I decided to see if the lorazepam Dr. Earvolino insisted I try would help.

I stared at a little white tablet that was about an eighth of an inch in diameter. I was supposed to take half of the tablet unless I needed full strength. I showed it to Chris.

"How am I supposed to cut something this tiny?"

I carefully positioned the tablet in a pill-cutter and pushed down. The result was one half-sized piece and crumbs. I wet my finger, picked up the crumbs and transferred them to my tongue, returning the half-tablet to the pill bottle for the next time I needed it.

The lorazepam did help. Soon I was able to concentrate on other matters.

CHAPTER 12
Life Before Cancer: Homeowners, 1968

After saving for a few years, Frank and I realized that home prices were going up faster than our income. The only way we would ever be able to buy a house was to plunge in and fix the price before it went up again. So, we took all we had saved, borrowed some money from my parents for a down payment, and bought a new three-bedroom, one-bath raised ranch house from a developer. The house would be built in a new subdivision in Tinley Park, a rapidly expanding middle-class suburb thirty miles from downtown Chicago.

Shortly before the builder was to break ground on our home, we got a call from our salesman, asking us to consider a change in the plan. When we arrived, he took us to a map that covered an office wall and showed all the lots in the development. He was smiling as he pointed to the location of the lot we had chosen.

"Here's the lot you bought," he said. "But this premium lot..." he moved his finger to a somewhat larger lot "...is available and I'd like to offer it to you instead. At no additional cost!" His grin widened.

I looked at Frank. His face was tight with anger. "Why would you do that? No one offers something for nothing. Be honest...what's wrong with that lot?"

I felt my face flush with embarrassment. I thought the salesman was a nice guy. Why was Frank suspicious?

The salesman's smile faded. "There's nothing wrong with the lot. It happens to be the best lot left. I can give it to you, and I thought it would make you happy. Look, why don't we drive over and see it?"

After viewing the lot, we realized it really was a substantial improvement over the one we had chosen. We accepted the man's offer. As I looked at Frank, his expression told me he was still leery, believing we had been talked into something that would backfire. We later found out that the man was retiring in a few days and wanted to remember his last home sale with a moment of generosity. To this day I regret that we ruined that experience for this kind man.

It wasn't that Frank did anything wrong, and perhaps I should have been more skeptical about the offer. But I prefer to assume that people are good and well-meaning until they prove otherwise. This experience showed me a side of Frank I hadn't noticed before, his belief that people were out to take advantage of him. I wasn't stupid enough to think that such people didn't exist—I just wanted to believe most people weren't like that.

However, buying a home when we did may have been a stretch. We couldn't afford a garage and started with hand-me-down furniture. But we made it happen, although buying food and paying bills was a week-to-week struggle.

I think it must have been during this time that I developed a lifelong sense of responsibility. Not only was I in charge of my sons, my home, and keeping my husband happy, but I was learning that my family and friends leaned on me too. I was a good listener, I had a good grasp of all sides of a problem, and I gave good advice. I also hated to say no or to be left out. I always made myself available when needed. But these traits put a limit on personal time.

Additionally, I was soon to add the burdens of contributing to our family income and running a medical practice. I didn't realize at the time that responsibility, although admittedly it gave me pleasure and pride, would turn into lifelong obligations I couldn't seem to escape.

CHAPTER 13
Getting Ready
December 26, 2017 through January 1, 2018

"Dolly and I researched from the clinical side and passed that information on to you because we knew you were worried. We wanted to be sure to share the optimistic outlook. We saw our role as providing you with guidance, helping with decision-making, choosing your treatment options." - Bob, son

"Why don't you read about tongue cancer online?" Chris asked. I think he must have noticed the anxious look on my face as I sat in our family room, thumbing once again through the binder I had gotten from oncology.

I understood he was trying to be helpful, but I didn't want to come across information that would make me doubt my medical team, nor did I want to confuse myself with more problems than I'd already thought about on my own. I could have looked up videos of procedures on YouTube too, but I didn't do that either. I was worried that too much detail would be scary rather than reassuring. It had taken some doing—and lorazepam crumbs—to get to the point that I could think calmly and logically.

One section in the binder listed the medical team, including their contact information. Another section described what would happen in the treatment room, side effects, what monitoring tests I would have, exams, support groups, nutrition, and more.

I looked at the list of support groups, but no group was specific for head and neck cancer, and not one was close to Lemont. In any case, I tended to be a private, do-it-myself kind of person. It was good to know the groups existed, but I doubted I'd be visiting any of them. If my cancer happened during or after COVID, I might have made a different decision, since many of these groups must have developed ways to meet virtually.

I would have liked to talk person-to-person with someone else who was either having the same treatment or had recently recovered from tongue cancer. That never happened. The reason I'm writing this memoir is to make that information available to help others.

To tone my body as much as I could before therapy started, I walked regularly thirty minutes a day on an indoor track at our park district. I had always hated exercise. In fact, I placed a cartoon on a tack board on my desk that expressed my feelings about working out. The Devil was speaking to a group of new arrivals to the fires of Hell. A balloon emerging from the Devil's mouth said, "We start with exercise."

I made exercise a priority and was faithful to my walk schedule.

Some friends suggested alternative or non-traditional medicine, and some of those options were covered in the binder: acupuncture, hypnosis, biofeedback, relaxation therapy, and more. But those weren't for me. All my years of working with top medical care providers had convinced me that traditional medicine was the best option for a cure.

Now God had a new place in my life. I was not a strongly religious person and went to Mass only occasionally.

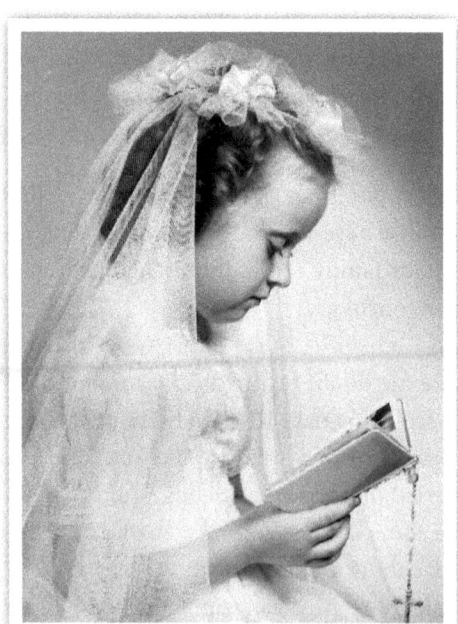

My First Holy Communion, age 6, with the blue crystal rosary

I belonged to St. James at Sag Bridge Church, though, and supported the parish. But throughout my life, when things got tough, I asked God for help.

At first, my Catholic guilt tortured me. Was I being punished? Had I done something that caused this disease? I ran through every little sin I could remember committing, wondering if that was the one that needed punishment. Then I searched in a drawer of family memorabilia and located the pale-blue crystal rosary I had received when I made my First Communion as a six-year-old.

I slipped the rosary under my pillow so it would be handy when I couldn't sleep. When I was awake tossing and turning, I said the rosary and called on God and the saints for help. St. Peregrine, the patron saint of cancer. St. Blaise, the patron of throat disease. Mary, of course. St. Patrick, my patron saint. And St. Jude, the patron of impossible causes.

So, having prepared myself medically, emotionally, and spiritually, I turned to practical matters. Then I started to panic about whether, with so few days remaining before treatment began, I had enough time to get everything done.

How many times had I seen on TV where someone was given bad news by his doctor and told to start getting his personal affairs in order? I hadn't been told that, but it wasn't my nature to leave important matters unfinished, and so little time remained. What if I forgot something important? If things didn't go well, it could be my last chance. Even if all went well, I couldn't know when I would be able to get back to certain projects and tasks.

What did "getting affairs in order" even mean? I'd never asked myself that before.

Fortunately, Chris and I had executed wills and powers of attorney some years ago. So I started by making lists of tasks that had to be done before I started treatment, and on separate pages projects that could wait and those I thought I'd be able to continue to do.

Just in case my disease didn't turn out well.

I organized our finances first. I thought I'd be able to continue to pay routine bills on time. I brought all our assets and accounts up to date and made a list of their locations, amounts, and applicable dates. I gave a copy to Chris. I called John and told him where to find all the information.

Taxes would be due April 15, and our accountant needed information from us before then to prepare them. I marked investment and tax obligations on a calendar and assembled documents in a folder so I wouldn't have to waste time searching for them if I didn't feel well enough when they were due.

Next, I sent regrets for a wedding and a graduation party we had planned to attend. I bought cards for all birthdays coming up in the next six months. I wouldn't be able to shop, so a card and a check would have to do this year. It would be best to stay away from people until my immune system recovered.

I canceled plans for a family vacation.

I had regular responsibilities to the Downers Grove Choral Society, the Lemont Library, and the Lemont Historical Society. I gathered all current and pending materials for each organization, wrote and printed out instructions, and met with people who would carry on my work during my absence.

As a writer, I had obligations for speaking engagements, signings, and other appearances. Medical appointments would soon fill my calendar instead. Since my energy level, appearance, and ability to handle side effects were unknown, I had no idea when I would be able to reschedule these appointments, so I canceled them indefinitely. I would have to disappoint some people.

I could have left some of these details to Chris, of course. He would have been more than willing to take care of home and family matters, and I could always "supervise" instead.

I guess in the end the reasons I worked through my list myself had a lot to do with my nature. Used to being "boss" in most situations, I saw myself moving into a role I found foreign. What happens when the person everyone counts on becomes dependent herself?

And what do you do when you're unsure about your future? There were things I felt compelled to do personally, other things I didn't have to do but preferred to do. Chris already did a lot and would be even busier taking care of me. I was in a place where not only was I in a position to take some matters off his plate, I also knew if I did everything myself I wouldn't get annoyed later about the way things were done.

Word of my cancer had gotten out, and gifts began to arrive from friends and family, cards and comfort items: soft pajamas, fuzzy slippers, wraps, pillows, a carry-all for daily trips to the hospital. It seemed people were envisioning me as in bed or housebound, but it was heartening to know that so many people cared and went out of their way to wish me well.

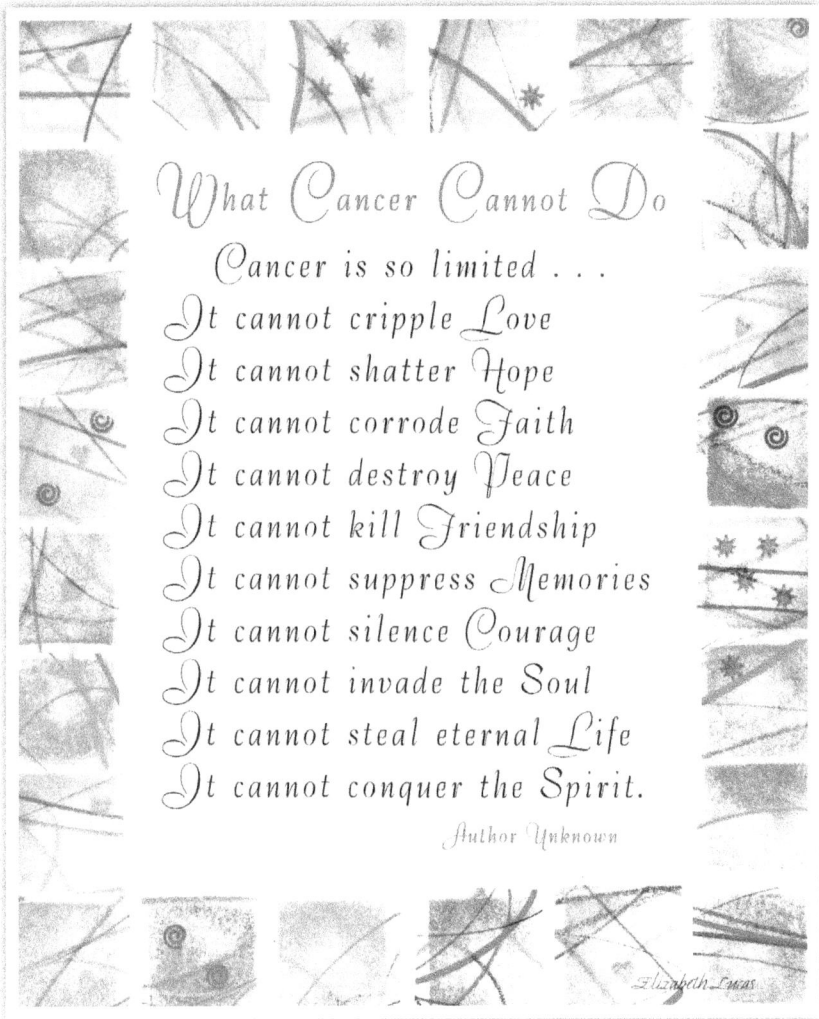

My friend, Sue, stopped by with a plaque titled "What Cancer Cannot Do." I put the plaque on the shelf over my fireplace, where I could see it every day.

The last day before I went for surgery I spent food shopping. It could be a long time before I'd be able to do that. The freezer and cabinets had to have food I'd be able to eat when I had no appetite and my mouth was sore. And there had to be food Chris liked to eat, since there would be days I couldn't cook for him. I was going to be dependent on Chris. The least I could do was be sure he ate well, even if I couldn't prepare the meals myself.

That same day I had my hair cut short. I wouldn't always have patience to fix my hair. I thought hair on my neck would aggravate the radiation burns I expected, and I might lose some hair anyway.

I finished all of this with some time to spare. That would have been impossible if I had been too sick or had to start treatment immediately.

I couldn't deny that this flurry of activity had another benefit. It kept me too busy to dwell on my medical problems and gave me a sense of accomplishment. And I was so tired by night that I fell into a deep sleep.

The last evening before my surgery I made one more trip into my home office. I gathered all the research notes, printed files, and other reference materials that had accumulated for the book I had been writing before I was diagnosed with cancer. I saved the uncompleted manuscript of *The Mystery at Mount Forest Island,* my third novel, to a flash drive and an external back-up drive. It was likely to be quite some time until I'd have the energy or the focus that writing a novel demanded. If that turned out to be the case, I had to be sure I could pick up where I left off once this was all over.

Had I thought of everything? Probably not. Time would tell.

I thought I was prepared, all my ducks in a row and my emotions under control. It was time to put my life on hold with only one thing to do—battle cancer.

PART TWO

Treating Cancer

CHAPTER 14
Biopsy
Tuesday, January 2, 2018

"I wanted to support you, take care of you, make sure you're okay, drive you to the hospital, all those things. Talk to the doctor. Of course, you did most of the talking..." - Chris, husband

Early in the morning on January 2, Chris drove me to Rush for the biopsy of the lesion on my tongue. Despite rush hour traffic, we arrived at the hospital by 9:15. The surgery was scheduled for 11:15. Afterward I would spend a few hours in recovery, and, providing no complications, I would go home that evening.

The biopsy was necessary to get detailed information about the tumor at the base of my tongue. We knew cancer had spread to my neck, but we didn't have details about the site where the cancer originated, called the primary lesion. It was likely, but not certain, that this was the area on my tongue seen on x-ray studies and during Dr. Thomas's laryngoscopy.

Dr. Thomas's examination under anesthesia would confirm the diagnosis with a detailed description of the appearance and location of the tumor, and pieces of the lesion would be removed and sent for exact pathological information. These details would be used to plan my radiation and chemotherapy.

I wasn't exceptionally nervous that morning. Having worked so long with surgeons, I was comfortable with the *idea* of surgery. I was having a minor procedure, similar to other surgeries I'd had under conscious, or mild, sedation. I didn't anticipate any complications. This time, though, I would be under general anesthesia, which was a bigger deal. But I expected to wake up with only a mild sore throat from the area where the biopsy was taken and from the tube passed down my throat by the anesthetist.

An assistant brought Chris and me into the preparation area, which looked much like the exam spaces in a typical emergency room: a stretcher, topped with a four-inch black cushion, in the middle of the room; a side chair; lots of medical equipment and monitors; oxygen on one wall and another wall curtained off from the hallway.

I took off my clothes and put on a hospital gown. A nurse took my vital signs and entered the results into a computer she had wheeled into the room. She put an IV in my arm. Then an ENT fellow came into the room to talk to me.

Rush is a teaching hospital. This means that medical students, interns, residents, and fellows (doctors in their final years of training in a medical specialty) are all involved in patient care. Typically, a person at one of these levels will examine a patient and take their history first, then discuss his opinions with the "attending," or staff doctor. I was not surprised to be seen by a fellow.

Some patients are annoyed when they have multiple doctors. They have already told their story to their personal doctor, and then repeated the story to a nurse, and then again to another person whose role they don't clearly understand, and they have yet to see their surgeon. I, however, was used to having students and residents involved in my care. I enjoyed talking with them and usually asked questions about their future plans.

The fellow told me he was almost finished with his training and would soon be taking boards, the examination that allows a doctor to practice in an area of specialty. I thought he was going to be an excellent doctor. He was not only thorough and knowledgeable, but he treated me with respect and compassion and actually appeared interested in what I had to say. Those qualities are valuable assets for a young doctor.

I expressed my concern about vomiting after surgery, explaining that had happened to me previously.

He said, "I'll talk to the anesthetist about that. It's most likely your vomiting was caused by a particular anesthetic agent. He can avoid using any of the likely culprits."

After he left, I expected a long wait, but was surprised when an assistant came into the room for me right away. Chris leaned over and kissed me as I lay on the cart, squeezed my arm and said, "See you soon." He gave me a big smile, but I noticed the edges of his cheeks were shaking.

When the technician wheeled me into the operating room, I had little time to worry or even think. Lying on the table on my back with bright lights above me on the ceiling, there seemed to be people all around me. Everyone was busy at something or other, handling a variety of instruments, tubes, and wires. I heard clicks, ticks, and whooshing sounds. The busyness all seemed rather chaotic, but everyone acted calm and purposeful, appearing to know exactly what to do.

The anesthetist introduced himself and asked if I had any questions. Over the clamor in the room, I repeated my concern about vomiting.

"Yes, we're aware of that. That's why we're putting this scopolamine patch behind your ear. The anesthetic you're getting doesn't usually cause vomiting, but the patch will give you more protection." He peeled the plastic off a small patch and placed it behind my left ear.

Dr. Thomas appeared on my right side. He squeezed my arm too.

"This is going to be over before you know it. How are you doing so far?"

"Fine, I guess," I said, wishing the surgery was over already. Maybe I wasn't as calm as I thought. I swallowed nervously and repeatedly, wondering how long it would be before I could swallow effortlessly and without pain again.

The medical team continued to bustle around me, and the next thing I knew I was waking up.

So, I'm done. It's all over.

I was still lying on a cart, too sleepy to open my eyes, but I heard people moving around and talking. My mouth was filled with secretions. I could swallow, but some remained and my mouth immediately filled again. I needed help. I called out, but no one came. I heard people nearby, walking around busily and talking, but they didn't answer me. *Why can't they hear me?*

In my groggy state I was more puzzled than panicky. I fell asleep again, and when I woke there was a nurse at my side.

"You're doing fine," she said. "Can I get you anything?"

"My mouth is full of saliva," I said. "I can't get rid of it all." The words came out blubbery.

She handed me a wad of tissues, and I pulled all the thick and abundant saliva I could out of my mouth. It instantly filled up again. She placed a full box of tissues beside my hand. As soon as I filled one tissue, I had to grab another one. The saliva was so annoying I forgot to be grateful that I wasn't vomiting. The secretions were a highly unpleasant surprise. I didn't know then that they were a sign of things to come.

As I became more and more aware of my surroundings, I realized that the reason the nurses didn't hear me when I first woke up wasn't because they were ignoring me, but because I only imagined I was calling them.

Somewhere along the line Chris came in, smiling, appearing relieved. He leaned over to kiss my cheek, held my hand, and then sat in a chair next to my cart.

"Dr. Thomas told me you did fine. They found exactly what they expected to. He said all is going perfectly."

I was glad to hear that, but I could think of little else except the gunk in my mouth. I was happy that there were no new problems. However, I was mildly annoyed by Chris's smile.

Can't he see how distressing these secretions are? He could probably tell I wasn't in noticeable pain, though.

Chris sat at my side while I filled tissue after tissue for the next two hours. Finally, the thick secretions diminished, and the nurse suggested it would help if I had something to eat. She brought me some apple juice.

I was a little afraid to drink anything, expecting pain when I swallowed. Surprisingly, the juice went down easily with little discomfort. I did feel better. I asked for a second carton.

I left the hospital about four that same evening. At home I was able to eat a small omelet. I had sharp pain when I swallowed solid food, but it wasn't worse than some sore throats I'd had. I was able to swallow my medications at bedtime without difficulty.

I was encouraged. This wasn't so bad. I could do this.

The first step to curing my cancer was over and all was going well thus far. The next day would be another full day, as long as this one. I had an appointment in oncology for my first infusion, and another in radiation oncology for simulation and staging. I wasn't clear about what simulation and staging was all about. I didn't think it was scary though. On the other hand, I knew that my infusion would have me sitting in a chair with a line running medicine into my arm. Anything could happen, and it could be nasty.

My treatment had begun. I felt like I was on a fast train to the vast unknown.

CHAPTER 15
Life Before Cancer: Working Mom, 1970

During the years I spent at home, I thought idly about returning to school someday to get a medical degree. In the late 1960s it was extremely difficult for women to be accepted into medical schools. A girl from my class who had graduated with a top GPA had given up after being turned down by school after school. It might be easier once my sons were in school. Perhaps I would try then. However, life interfered with that possibility and the opportunity never developed.

Frank's company made some cuts, and he was out of work. He was unable to find a job at first, and the job he eventually found didn't pay all our bills, so I jumped at an opportunity I was offered to manage a small medical clinic fifteen minutes from home. True, I wasn't fulfilling my dream of being a doctor, but I had a foot in the door. Maybe things would change.

So, in 1970 I began my career as administrator of a small medical group, taking administrative courses and learning what I was doing on the job. I was twenty-eight at the time. John was four years old, and Bob was three. I stayed with them most of the day and worked evenings, leaving the house after Frank got home to be with them.

Until I started thinking about medical school, I had never had any interest in, nor demonstrated an aptitude for, any type of service career. Yet it turned *out I had a knack for medical administration, and I loved what I did.*

Falling into the position of being a "boss" seemed natural to me. I was already running my home and to some extent the lives of my family and friends. I liked the freedom of making my own decisions and the pride in seeing them turn out well. I remembered my childhood years when I got so much enjoyment out of "playing teacher," and realized that the skills and talents that made that game so enjoyable were similar to what I was doing at work.

Few administrators have a background in medicine, but my degree in biology gave me an understanding and appreciation of what the doctors I worked for did. I was fortunate enough to work with outstanding surgeons—always surgeons—some of the best in the world. My career in the medical field was to last forty years, the last fifteen spent at Rush University Medical Center.

I got used to being in charge. Organizational skills, recognizing problems and making informed decisions, and running the office seemed to come naturally to me. At the same time, I was beginning to get a glimpse of what this assumed responsibility meant.

CHAPTER 16
Chemotherapy Begins - Second Day of Treatment
Wednesday Morning, January 3, 2018

"We wished we could be there, because although the treatment is very effective it is physically and emotionally very hard. I see it all the time. There is toxicity and difficulty handling normal activities. My patients need support at home." - Dolly, daughter-in-law

"I was very thankful that we weren't far away if you needed something. You had a good husband." - Clare, daughter-in-law

My daughter-in-law Dolly said she advised her oncology patients to start out with a substantial breakfast on the morning of their first infusion—and to prepare for a long day. She reminded me I would be bouncing from the Professional Building, where the oncology offices were, to radiation therapy across the street in one of the main hospital buildings, and back, with each appointment taking substantial time.

Unlike most people who gain weight over the holidays, I had lost five pounds—from anxiety, not from cancer. I lose my appetite when I get nervous, and once I found out I had cancer I didn't feel like eating at all. However, that morning I forced myself to down a bowl of oatmeal. I didn't know then that oatmeal was a sign of things to come—hot cereal turned out to be one of the few foods I could tolerate when my appetite deserted me.

I showered and brushed my teeth, blew my hair dry, and applied eye makeup and light lipstick. Once again, I dressed carefully in comfortable but professional-looking clothes that were warm and easy to change in and out of. I believed it made a difference to my care team. If I took care with my appearance, they would treat me with respect.

Never sure how long the thirty-mile trip to Rush would take, Chris and I left the house at 8:15 that morning for my ten o'clock appointment. When we arrived in the oncology department, I was directed to a kiosk at the front of the room. A sign at the kiosk read, "Take a number and have a seat until registration calls your number." I noticed a box of masks next to the kiosk.

"Should I wear one of these?" I asked the person at the information desk.

"Not unless you're sick," the assistant said. "They're to keep you from spreading infection to other patients."

"Oh," I said, feeling a bit dumb.

This was, of course, several years before COVID, which prompted a new way of life with its worldwide restrictions and controversies that included the commonplace use of masks.

I didn't take a mask but, not wanting to catch something from someone either, Chris and I chose seats as far as possible from other patients in the large, L-shaped reception room. The center of the L had a row of ten registration desks with chairs in front of each.

The waiting area was filled with an assortment of cushioned seats and looked like it could hold about seventy-five people. That morning it was about half full. I studied the people as I waited, sorting out patients from those that accompanied them. Two patients were seated in wheelchairs, a few had walkers, but most were ambulatory and getting around normally. One woman was curled up on a sofa, clearly ill. Not many of the patients looked sick, and only a few wore masks. I didn't see anyone with a rash.

I leaned over and whispered to Chris. "Most of these patients don't look sick. I think that's a good sign, don't you?"

He nodded.

"When I worked across from oncology," I whispered, "I saw cancer patients all the time. It got so I could spot wigs pretty well. It made me wonder why cancer patients all seemed to wear bad wigs that were so obvious. I don't see many today though. Either fewer patients are losing hair or more are getting better wigs now."

"How could you tell?"

"Oh, it didn't fit right. You've seen bad wigs, I'm sure. Too big or covered too much forehead. Wrong color. Bad style. Fake-looking. How sad to be sick and think people are staring at you. Sorry to say, I could have been one of those staring people. Now I have to wonder if soon I'll be the one being stared at."

Before he could comment, I heard my number called. I went to the registration desk, where a friendly man confirmed my appointment, asked me a few questions, and typed on a keyboard. Then he attached a plastic identification bracelet to my wrist, handed some papers to me, and smiled.

"Take a seat. A nurse will call your number soon. Give her these papers."

At first, I was a bit put off that numbers were used instead of names. Then I remembered that HIPAA, the national law that defines patient privacy rules, discourages the use of names, especially in waiting areas. What if, for instance, Michelle Obama or Brad Pitt were to be called? The world would know before their appointment was over. No one wants his cancer to be broadcast publicly.

Again, I waited only a few minutes. A staff member took Chris and me to an exam room in the same area my initial consultation had taken place. She took my vital signs: weight, temperature, oxygen, and blood pressure.

"As soon as you arrive every week," the assistant said, "the lab will do a blood count, blood chemistry panel, and magnesium level, since Cetuximab depletes magnesium. Today we already have baseline tests from when you were here for your consultation, so we only need your vital signs.

"Each time you come, your blood test results and your vitals are sent down to the pharmacy. Dr. Fidler and the pharmacist make decisions based on those results to calculate and mix your infusion. After you see our nurse and your oncologist, you'll go over to radiation oncology for your treatment, and while you're there, the pharmacist will be getting your infusion ready. Then you'll come back here, have your infusion, and then you'll go home. Do you have any questions?"

I did, but I thought I'd wait to ask my nurse or doctor. So I smiled and shook my head.

As she was leaving the room, Mandy, the clinical coordinator, and a short, slender woman in her twenties entered the room together. The young woman introduced herself as Mary, the head and neck oncology nurse practitioner.

"Good," Mary said, noticing the white plastic binder in my lap. "You brought your folder like we asked you to. Let's go over it and answer any questions you might have."

I was glad I hadn't taken the assistant's time earlier. I'd remember to hold questions unless I wanted a range of opinions on a particular matter.

Mary opened the binder and went over each section, asking if I understood what I read there. I nodded each time. Then she handed me two brochures published by the American Cancer Society: "Chemotherapy: What It Is, How It Helps" and "If You Have Head or Neck Cancer."

"These might be helpful," she said.

Since my tumor was at the base of my tongue, I was particularly worried about how my ability to swallow was going to be affected.

"My mother…um…" I began, stopped, then started again. "My mother had a stroke and spent years with a feeding tube. I want to do everything I can to avoid that."

Mary's eyes softened. "We can't promise. It will help if you're religious about mouth care, swallowing exercises, and nutrition. But if you lose too much weight, I'm afraid you'll have to have a tube. Most people are able to get off the tube when they start eating well again. You'll have a speech therapist and a nutritionist. They'll both help you, and all of us will do our best."

She meant to reassure me, but I found her words alarming. *Some people don't get off the tube?* "But I don't have an appetite *now*, and we haven't even started. I've lost ten pounds, five in the last week. And if the chemo makes me nauseous…"

I stopped, realizing my own words were justifying a feeding tube. I felt my cheeks quiver and a sudden ache in my stomach. How would I get through chemotherapy if I was nauseous for months? What was going to happen when my body went to war with my disease? Yes, I know I was fixated on that concern. My oncologists didn't know me yet, didn't know how easily my stomach was upset, how I expected to be even sicker when chemo and radiation would change the way things tasted and my mouth was dry and sticky.

What if I get so sick I can't finish my cancer treatment? Does my cancer take over then and I die? No, that won't happen—don't think about that now.

"Remember," Mary reminded me, "Cetuximab is not actually a chemotherapy agent, but a monoclonal antibody that works with your immune system to kill cancer cells. This drug doesn't have the extreme side effects you expect." She patted my arm. "In any event, if you do experience nausea or vomiting, we have medicine for that. You're going to be fine."

Altogether, I spent about forty minutes chatting with Mary and exchanging information. I made a lot of notes in the binder. Then she examined me and entered information in the computer.

Mary paused at the door. "You'll be glad to know that your treatment will be finished before Dr. Fidler goes on leave."

I gave her a blank look. "On leave?"

She grinned. "I thought you would've noticed that she's pregnant. A little boy. She has another little boy at home now."

She would have two boys. Just like me.

Dr. Fidler's visit was short. She greeted me pleasantly, felt my pulse and neck, examined my mouth, and listened to my chest. Then she sat down at the computer and made some additional notes.

"I know you're worried about nausea. Let's not wait until it happens. I'll write you a prescription now that you can take at the first sign. I'm also writing for an antibiotic to have on hand if you need it and something for a skin rash in case of allergy. Is Walgreens still your pharmacy? Do you want to fill your prescription there or through our outpatient pharmacy?"

"Walgreens, please."

She got up and put her hand over mine. "You're ideal for this study. You're going to do well."

After she left the room, I exchanged a glance with Chris. "Everyone keeps saying I'm going to do well. Do they mean that, or are they just being encouraging?"

He retrieved my coat from a hook on the door and spread it open for me. "I'm sure they want to be encouraging, but I also think in your case they mean it. As they said, you have every reason to do well." He shook my coat, since I'd made no move to put it on yet. "Now, let's get on over to radiation therapy."

I slipped my arms into my coat sleeves. I had to get over this fear of vomiting. Everything I'd experienced so far had been reassuring and not very scary, but I knew I had to do my part if I wanted to make my next few months easier. My medical team was knowledgeable, understanding, patient, and compassionate. I was encouraged by that and fully intended to follow every instruction to the letter. I wanted to survive, but I also wanted to limit my side effects—especially that feeding tube.

If the worst happened, it wouldn't be because of something I should have done but didn't!

CHAPTER 17
Radiation Simulation
Same Day –
Wednesday, January 3, 2018 – Late Morning

"Dr. Layan talked about a hospital in Texas—a doctor he knew—that gave us another option that had good cure rates. We couldn't know if it would work or not, but he gave us hope." - Chris, husband

Dolly had been right about the long day. It wasn't even noon yet, and I still had to face radiation therapy, and my first infusion wouldn't be until mid-afternoon. Already I wanted to be home, and the infusion, the part that scared me, hadn't even begun. The surgery the previous day hadn't been bad, and all we'd done so far this day was talk, but stress was taking its toll.

Radiation therapy was entered directly from its own small parking area. One of two receptionists, Sheryl, a pleasant middle-aged woman sitting beside a man in wire-rimmed glasses who appeared to be about thirty, greeted us and verified my appointment time.

"You can have a seat in the waiting area." She pointed to a room open to the reception desk. "Since this is your first day, someone will come out to get you. Did you park in the garage?"

I told her we did.

She handed me a card. "Here's a parking pass. Next time you come, put this pass in the front window of your car, and park anywhere you can find a space out there. You won't have to pay parking, not even the discounted patient rate."

That was a surprise. I had expected to pay the $8.00 patient rate for every visit for the thirty-five visits scheduled. Little things like that mattered.

The radiation therapy waiting area was much smaller than oncology, seating about thirty people, with cushioned chairs on every wall and two rows of seats in the center. We selected chairs in a corner where I could watch people coming and going. About half the room was filled. Everyone seemed reasonably healthy. One wall was all windows covered by closed blinds; on another wall, a large-screen television ran a news show.

Almost immediately I heard a loudspeaker. "Mr. Carney, you can go back now." A middle-aged man got up and walked out, turning a corner after he left the room. I noted the use of a name instead of a number and wondered why.

I leaned over to Chris and whispered, "I guess he knows his way around."

The automatic doors to the parking lot opened into the reception area, and two paramedics pushed in a large woman on a stretcher, accompanied by another large woman. The woman on the stretcher appeared to be partly conscious and moaning. The paramedics checked with the receptionist and then rolled the stretcher into the waiting room. They paid little attention to the patient, but spoke to her friend, who was already complaining about waiting.

My gaze met Chris's. Was that going to be me a month from now? Maybe the woman was sick for other reasons or hadn't caught her disease early. Before I could observe any more, a large man in his mid-thirties came through a doorway on the opposite side of the reception area, entered the waiting room, and called "Mrs. Camalliere."

Chris and I stood up. "Can my husband come with me?" I asked.

He shook his head. "Sorry. Only patients can go back into the department."

Chris took my purse and coat, gave me a hug and a peck on the cheek, whispered, "Good luck," and returned to his seat.

"I'm Robbie," the man said. "I'm Dr. Layan's nurse." Although he was tall and hefty like a football player, he reminded me more of a teddy bear once I heard his soft-spoken voice and noticed his kind smile.

Robbie took me into an exam room and checked my vitals again. I sat in a chair while he gave me an introduction to the department. This included another American Cancer Society pamphlet, "Radiation Therapy, What It Is, How It Helps" and a brochure welcoming me to Rush University Medical Center Radiation Treatment.

Robbie explained the radiation side effects I should expect: skin changes, changes in taste, mouth sores, dry mouth, decreased appetite, fatigue, and so on. He told me how to reach him and invited me to contact him with questions. He gave me a bottle of medication called MuGard, which he said was to help with my mouth symptoms, and a skin lotion.

"We get samples from the pharmaceutical firms," he said. "Let me know if you need more or if these don't work. We may be able to give you others that will work better." Again, I was surprised. Free parking, and now free drugs! Cool.

Then Dr. Layan came into the room and explained the procedure. The task for the day was to map the areas that would be treated.

"The challenge of radiation therapy is to kill all existing cancer cells while harming as little as possible the normal, healthy cells," he said. "This is very important for cancers in the head and neck, since there are many vital structures in the area that need to retain normal function if possible. Think about everything that happens in the mouth, throat, and neck—the areas that will be radiated."

I knew much of what he would say next, because of my long career in the medical field and because I had reviewed the anatomy after I knew I had cancer.

"The mouth contains not only teeth and tongue, but also gums, mucous membranes, salivary glands, bones of the lower face and jaw, muscles, blood supply, and nerves." As he spoke, he held up his hand and counted off each structure. "The tongue determines how food tastes, and the salivary glands produce a fluid that mixes with food during the chewing process to prepare it to be swallowed as a ball, or bolus. The tongue is also involved in speech, chewing, and swallowing." He stopped and looked at me to see if I was following him.

I was. None of what he mentioned were structures I wanted to do without.

During my recent review of anatomy, I also understood that the neck connects the head to the rest of the body, providing pathways for circulation, nerves, breathing, and digestion. Major arteries and veins pass from the chest through the neck to supply circulation to the head, feeding the brain. Major nerves, including the cranial nerves, control sensation, movement, and organ functions in the head and neck, such as hearing, smell, and taste. Lymph nodes and ducts are along the cervical spine, face, and jaw. The neck also contains muscles, bones, skin, and thyroid and parathyroid glands.

In the throat, or lower neck, the pharynx connects the mouth to both the lungs and the esophagus, separated by a muscle, the epiglottis, which shuts during swallowing to prevent food from aspirating into the lungs. The larynx, or voice box, needed for speech, is in the lower neck.

Bottom line, the neck is pretty darn important.

Dr. Layan explained that my primary tumor at the base of my tongue was in close proximity to many of these structures, including the taste buds, the salivary glands, and the epiglottis. I really wanted to be able to taste my food, have saliva, and be able to swallow safely. Some impairment during treatment was expected, but my targeted treatment would be tailored to allow most of the function to remain or return.

This was the benefit of the trial I had agreed to. If I had opted for standard radiation, I could have expected more serious effects.

Dr. Layan said, "To protect the vital areas in your neck that aren't involved in cancer, target areas will be identified, and radiation doses calculated and programmed into the radiology computers that will deliver your radiation. This will take the radiation dosimetrists, radiation physicists, and radiation oncologist about a week to do, so you won't receive any radiation today."

Now that I'd begun, I was anxious to keep going. "But it's already been two weeks since we talked about this. I have to wait another week?"

"One week won't make a difference. It's also critically important that you remain motionless throughout the procedure. You'll wear a mask that will immobilize you. We'll make your mask today, and we'll also take a baseline CT scan that will be used in the calculations."

I had no clue what the calculations involved, but the process *sounded* impressive, with all those people studying a variety of factors and coming up with something so precise. But the mask was a little concerning. I had never had an attack of claustrophobia, but I didn't like the idea of being tied down and unable to move if I felt the urge. But I was also a squirmer, so if keeping still was so important, I'd appreciate the help.

Then Robbie led me to a changing room and asked me to take off everything above my waist and put on a hospital gown. After changing, I followed him to the treatment room. The hallway opened into a corridor with two doors. On the right, a room with a long counter that ran from one end to the other was filled with monitors and keyboards and technical equipment. Two people, busy at their desks, stood up and came out to meet me.

Robbie introduced me to my treatment team.

Vani was a short, slightly plump, dark-skinned woman who appeared to be in her fifties with warm brown eyes and a Middle Eastern accent. She seemed quiet and pleasant. Paul was a large, attractive, prematurely balding, thirty-something Caucasian man, outgoing, enthusiastic, and energetic. Paul was the talker, I immediately decided. Vani the comforter.

They led me through the other door into the treatment room.

"It looks like a scanner," I said, gazing at the huge white donut that dominated the center of the room. Vani helped me sit on the side of the long table that slid in and out of the donut, like the CT scanner and the PET scanner I was already familiar with.

"It *is* a scanner," Paul said, standing with his hands in the pockets of his white lab coat. "But it also delivers your radiation. We control everything from that room you saw us sitting in.

"Today we're going to do another scan, which will be used to program the doses of radiation you'll receive. Then we're going to make your mask."

"Yes, that's what Dr. Layan told me."

"Dr. Layan is the best," Paul said. "You're in good hands." Again, the reassurance, but I was glad to hear it, especially since his comment came unprompted from someone in a position to know, and not as a result of a question from me.

He asked me to lie on the table and adjusted my position. Once satisfied, he said, "I'll be in the control room. You won't be able to see us, but we'll be watching you every moment on monitors and will talk to you over a speaker. It's important to hold absolutely still when the scanner is operating. We'll tell you when to stop moving or breathing. If you need anything, hold up a hand. We'll see you, stop the procedure, and come to talk to you. Ready?"

I was ready. And, as I'd been told, the procedure seemed like other scans I'd already had. I stayed still, and there was no need to stop. After the scan, Paul and Vani came back into the room.

"You did good," Paul said, smiling. "Now let's get your mask made and get you out of here."

Still lying on my back on the table, I watched as Paul approached with what appeared to be a thirty-inch square sheet of flexible off-white plastic mesh. Vani asked me to close my eyes, and they placed the mesh over my head, shoulders, and upper torso. The plastic felt warm.

"Keep your eyes closed until we tell you," Vani said. The cooperative patient, I did as they said. I felt them pressing all over my head, face, shoulders, and chest as they molded the warm mesh to my body. It was tight. I could breathe normally, but Vani asked me not to move my mouth or eyelids until the mesh hardened. That only took a few minutes, since soon they pulled the mask away.

I looked at what they had made. The mask looked like off-white mesh, cast as the front half of a life-sized head-and-shoulders bust of a person. I didn't see any resemblance to me. It seemed rather generic, but they told me they would definitely know which mask was mine. The mask struck me as odd and perhaps even a bit spooky.

All of this was new and much of what happened behind the scenes was beyond my understanding, but the wonders of technology impressed me and immediately I felt I could trust this team. If anyone could cure my cancer, these were the right people.

It was time for the radiation team to do their work, and time for my first infusion of Cetuximab. The emotion, wealth of new information and experiences inspired confidence, but I felt tired, like I'd had enough excitement for the day. Unfortunately, the day still wasn't over yet. I retrieved Chris from the waiting room and dragged myself back across the street to medical oncology.

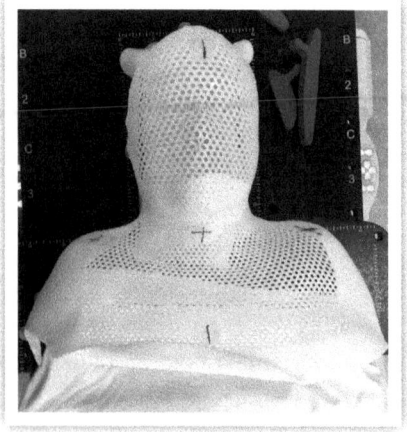

The mask.

CHAPTER 18

First Infusion
Same Day –
Wednesday, January 3, 2018 – Mid-Afternoon

"Of course, I was concerned. Initially your cancer was considered stage IV, and that's bad. Usually you don't survive stage IV cancer, but your cancer is an exception. It was later downgraded to stage III.

We were worried about whether treatment would be effective. Close to ninety percent of people who get your treatment regimen are cured, so that's really optimistic. And then, of course, the side effects—what's that going to be like? We were really happy you were able to get into the trial, because that saved you from excessive radiation. That's no fun." - Bob, son

After Chris and I sat for a short time in another typical waiting area, a nurse called my number and Chris and I followed her to the infusion room. I was about to begin the part of treatment that I dreaded most—the part that could make me sick to my stomach.

The room was divided into treatment stations that formed a semicircle around a long C-shaped nurses' desk. The nurse that greeted me called the stations "pods." Each station had a turquoise leather-like recliner with a desk-like arm, a straight-backed chair, a tall wooden supply cabinet, and a wheeled cart that held an infusion pump. I counted ten stations. Although the stations were separated, no patient had complete privacy, and each patient was always visible to the nurses.

Next to the nurses' desk was a more private room with sliding glass doors. My nurse led me there for my first infusion. Chris sat in a chair that looked semi-comfortable, and I seated myself on the recliner. After verifying my identity, running me through routine questions, and taking my vital signs yet again, the nurse offered me a pillow and a blanket, fresh from the warmer. I welcomed the offer at this point, as this was January in Chicago and every room I'd been in had been cold.

I watched somewhat uneasily as the nurse assembled an assortment of medication bottles, swabs, sealed plastic packages, and tubes. She used sanitizer on her hands and put on gloves. She selected a vein on the back of my right hand, scrubbed my skin with an alcohol wipe, and then inserted an intravenous cannula. The plastic tubing appeared flexible and very thin; I felt a slight prick when it punctured my skin. The tiny cannula that remained in my hand when she finished was only a little uncomfortable.

"I'm going to flush this now with a little saline," the nurse said, after taping the tubing in place. She pulled back on the syringe, and my blood flowed up the line, proving it was inserted and working properly. The saline she injected felt like a rush of cold water.

She left the room and returned in a few moments, rolling in a computer on a cart. She asked my name yet again and used a handheld scanner gun to transfer my wristband information into the computer. Then she scanned each bottle of medicine on the tray and turned to smile at me.

"We scan your band, your infusion, and all your pre-infusion medications so there's a record of everything you've been given."

I exchanged glances with Chris. We were glad to know every precaution was being taken to be sure I got what my doctors had prescribed.

The nurse kept talking in a friendly manner. "We refer to everything we do here as chemotherapy, administering agents that stop or slow the growth of cancer cells. Cetuximab, though, is a monoclonal antibody, which works along with your body's immune system to kill cancer cells."

I knew this already, but I nodded.

"Today we're going to give you what's called a "loading dose," she said. "It's double the dose you'll get for the rest of your infusions. Cetuximab stays in your body for a week, which also means it takes more time to reach therapeutic levels. So we give you a larger dose to start to get you to the desired level as soon as possible. You'll be here about three hours today."

I glanced at Chris again. My face probably showed my dismay. Three more hours! While walking over from the radiation oncology department I felt like I had regained some energy since that experience had gone so well. But now the thought of three more hours before I could go home almost brought tears to my eyes.

The nurse seemed to sense my disappointment. She placed a gloved hand on my shoulder. "The time will go fast. You can read or lie back in the recliner and sleep if you like—or chat with your husband. Or maybe he can go down and get you both some food if you haven't had lunch yet. It's okay to eat during the infusion." She looked in Chris's direction.

"Is it going to make me sick?" I asked.

"You shouldn't be sick while you're here. It takes a while for stomach distress to happen, and many people don't get sick at all."

"I get sick easy though—real easy," I said nervously.

"Yes, I read that in your chart. Right now, I'm going to give you a pre-infusion injection. It's a combination of Benadryl to prevent a possible allergic reaction and Decadron to boost the effect of Cetuximab. These drugs also help prevent nausea."

I was somewhat relieved, if not completely confident in the precautions. They were doing their best to deal with my problems. I couldn't blame them if their efforts didn't work. I'd have to wait and see what happened and deal with the consequences.

The injection was given through my cannula, so I wasn't stuck with another needle.

"We have to let the medications get into your system before we start the infusion. That'll take about half an hour. Call me if you need anything—you can see me at my desk right outside. Can I get you something first? How about some juice? Did you eat today?"

"Not since breakfast, but I'm not hungry." I made a face. "Nerves."

"I'm going to bring in some juice—drink it or not as you like. But you have to keep your strength up." She looked at Chris. "Perhaps your husband here can run down to the cafeteria and get you something," she said again. "Next week, bring a snack with you."

After she returned to her desk, leaving two small containers of orange juice, I handed one to Chris. "I'm going to save this until after she starts the infusion, I think. What are you going to do for three hours?"

He pulled the top off the juice, splashing a few drops on his pants. He brushed at the drops with his free hand, then sipped the juice. "I want to stay here until after she starts the infusion. Unless you want me to get you something…"

"It's going to be a long time. I might sleep or read…but you should eat. I don't want to have to worry about you too. Maybe I could handle some yogurt."

"Let's play it by ear," he said, reaching for my hand.

I dropped the back of the recliner halfway, raised my legs to level, adjusted the pillow, and closed my eyes. I sneaked a peek a few minutes later. Although both of our hands still rested, twined, on the side of the recliner, Chris's head was drooped, and his eyes were closed. "Let him sleep," I thought.

Alone then with my thoughts, I just wanted to get the infusion over with.

It wasn't until years later that I learned that at first my cancer was thought to be at Stage IV, but early in treatment downgraded to Stage III. I hadn't wanted to know, fearing it would color my approach to treating the disease. If it was too far advanced, I may have thought *what's the use* and given up. If it was too early, I may have thought treatment was less important. I knew that my cancer had spread to my lymphatic system and to my neck. That was enough to deal with at the time.

Stage III means that the cancer has spread to both the lymphatic system and to nearby tissues. Stage IV means the spread has involved more distant parts of the body. These stages define the treatment and the likelihood of success of the treatment. Although my cancer was at an advanced stage, my doctors felt that I fell into a class that had a ninety percent cure rate.

Today would indicate how well I'd be able to tolerate the medicine I needed to kill my cancer. What was I committing myself to? How sick would it make me? Would it be successful? Maybe I'd stay the course, but it wouldn't do any good.

Let's just get this started!

I didn't sleep, and Chris's nap was short, as the nurse soon interrupted.

"Ready?" she asked.

I nodded, my smile weak.

With everything in place, all she had to do was turn the little valve that released the infusion drip and watch the little vial below the connection to be sure the drip rate was correct.

"The infusion itself will take about an hour, perhaps a little longer. Then you have to stay here another hour while we monitor you, just to be sure you don't have a reaction."

She turned a little dial located on the clear plastic line that ran from the pump to my IV. We both watched as the first drips slowly fell into the little clear vial until the nurse seemed satisfied.

"The pump will beep when the infusion is done. We'll be checking anyway, but don't let the beep startle you." Two minutes later, she left the room, and Chris and I were alone again.

I kept turning my head toward the pump, watching the drip, every nerve on edge, waiting for my body to react in some way. I could see Chris glancing at the pump, and at me, frequently. Neither of us said anything, but he gave me one of those big, affectionate smiles that always make me feel like I'm not alone.

Oh God! Make this work! And please don't let me be sick!

As she had predicted, I didn't feel much as the Cetuximab slowly trickled into me—anything, in fact, except sleepy and a little lightheaded, and I figured I felt that way more due to nerves than an effect of the infusion.

It wasn't like Chris to ask how I felt. He knew I'd tell him if something was wrong, and he wouldn't want to increase my anxiety by asking me to define my problems. So, we just sat, silent for the most part. I could have asked Chris for the Kindle in my purse, but I didn't. I knew I wouldn't be able to concentrate.

Chris closed his eyes again. I knew he must be tired too, and he'd have to sit in a straight-backed chair for three whole hours.

"Why don't you go down and eat now?" I said.

"Maybe later, unless you want that yogurt."

"I'm good."

I took my phone from my pocket, checked e-mails, messages, and Facebook. Nothing needed attention. I looked at Chris. I didn't know how he could sleep upright, but he did, slumped in the chair. I could ask the nurse for a pillow for him too, but right now I didn't want to disturb him.

Feeling small and powerless, I closed my eyes and dozed.

When I awoke, the nurse was at my side, disconnecting the drip. Apparently, she arrived and stopped the infusion before the pump beeped. I had a painful urge to urinate. All that fluid, that I now viewed as *pouring* into my body instead of dripping, forced all other thoughts from my mind. I was glad I hadn't drunk the orange juice. Fortunately, the restroom was right next to my pod.

Chris and I waited the obligatory extra hour for observation, and then, just like that, my first chemotherapy was over. I felt nothing except tired and still sleepy despite the hours I had dozed in the recliner. It would take over an hour to get home in evening rush hour traffic. Once there, I probably still wouldn't want to eat, but would be very happy to put on a nightgown and get into my own bed. I felt exhausted but vastly relieved. I didn't get sick!

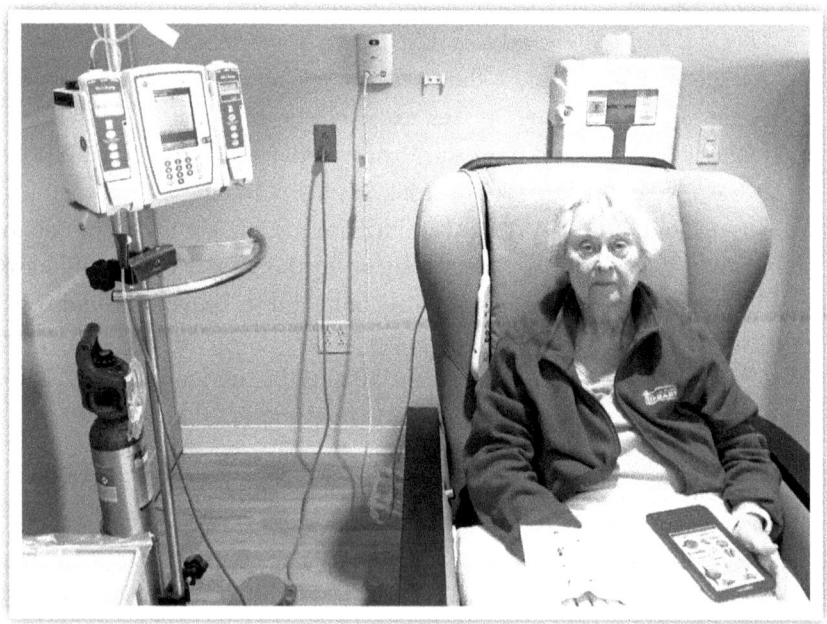

Me in "the pod."

CHAPTER 19
Life Before Cancer: Dependencies Grow, 1970-1980

*I*was beginning to realize that a lot of people depended on me. I was accepting commitments not only from my immediate family but from friends, coworkers, and patients that came to the office. I was a good listener, and it was hard for me to say no. People trusted me. It felt like a compliment.

One of these people was Bill, a good friend who owned a Jaguar dealership a half block from my office. We often got together on the spur of the moment at either my office or his to chat. Bill was tall and unusually thin, with a receding hairline and a neat mustache. He had a sarcastic sense of humor that I found entertaining. I was an idiot about cars, but Bill was always available when I needed advice on car matters, or even personal matters.

One day during a visit to my office Bill had a coughing spell. I didn't like what I heard.

"How long have you been coughing like that?" I asked after he controlled the spell.

"Too long," he said. "Over a month now."

"You haven't seen your doctor," I pointed out. Bill was a patient at our office, and I knew he hadn't been in.

"I suppose I should do that. To be honest, I've been unusually tired too."

"You smoke all day. How long has it been since you've had a chest x-ray?"

"Years. Lots of years." He didn't say anything for a time. Then he turned to me and asked, "Can you help me?"

I made a snap decision. Bill was there in my office and might make excuses and put off my advice if I let him leave. His doctor was at the hospital doing surgery and wouldn't be available for hours, and I had learned to take x-rays for our office. I knew his doctor would order a chest x-ray. I made the same decision for Bill as I'd make for any patient under the same circumstances.

I took Bill back to the x-ray room and took films of his chest. Even then our equipment was outdated. We still processed x-rays in a manual tank in our office. When I hung the film to dry over the developing tank, I studied it. Bill stood in the open darkroom doorway looking over my shoulder.

"How's it look?" he asked, sounding anxious.

At first Bill's film looked like a normal, thin male chest. His heart was normal in size, and his spine, ribs, and lung tissue were clear and well exposed. And then I noticed a fuzzy round spot about the size of a nickel. And then another one, a little smaller. And another. And another. I stopped counting. I felt a cold sensation in my stomach. What would I tell Bill?

I pointed at one of the spots—only one. "There's something a little unusual here. I don't know what it is, but I'll have your doctor see it as soon as he gets in."

I didn't know—for sure—what I saw. But I knew it wasn't good. I looked at chest films many times a week, and I'd never seen anything like that.

Bill went back to work with a worried look on his face, and I returned to my office where I let some tears fall. When his doctor arrived, he confirmed an obvious lung cancer, and we called Bill to come over right away to give him the result.

Over the next few days, Bill had more studies and was seen by a thoracic surgeon. Bill had heard about a surgeon at Mayo Clinic and wanted to see him but couldn't get an appointment. Could I help?

My first inquiries weren't any more successful than Bill's had been, but with persistence I was able to get through to a secretary at Mayo who found a spot in the schedule within a week. Bill was seen at Mayo and was operated on there. The surgery was painful, but successful. He had a gradual recovery and thereafter led a normal, cancer-free life for more than twenty years.

Bill's story was one of many. I began to realize that I had become the person people turned to for help, not only in my family but among my friends, and the person my employers, my employees, and some of our patients sought when they needed something.

Since childhood, I had always set aside personal interests, first to concentrate on educating myself, then becoming responsible for my family. Now in addition, I was a breadwinner and responsible for an office of five doctors, a lab, a staff of fourteen, and numerous patients, as well as obligations to friends.

Part of me would have felt guilty if I did less, and another part of me actually wanted the burden. I found responding to people's needs rewarding. Regardless, the situation left me no time for other interests. But that was all right then. I was young, and "my time" was surely in my future, if I worked hard first.

CHAPTER 20

The Evening After—Worries Accelerate
Thursday, January 4, 2018 – 2 a.m.

"It's hard to see people you love hurting." - John, son

"You were probably worrying too much, but it's your body, your cancer, so what would you expect? You didn't talk about it much and seemed to get along okay. You didn't complain much. But you worried." - Chris, husband

I awoke at two in the morning with a bad headache, extreme muscle weakness, and, yes, the nausea I had dreaded since I first learned I had cancer.

Damn it! I told them over and over I'd get sick! Why didn't anyone listen to me!

Furious, but not wanting to wake Chris, I wobbled to the bedroom table where I kept my medications, barely able to stand, fearing I'd collapse to the floor when the muscles in my legs gave out. Using the flashlight on my phone, I located the information that came with the pain medication I'd been prescribed but had no reason to take yet. As I suspected, tramadol sometimes caused nausea. My headache wasn't worse than others I'd survived with Tylenol, so I dragged myself into the bathroom and took two Tylenol instead, fearful of making my nausea worse.

I'd been told several times that my first dose was a loading dose, but I didn't give it too much thought. Now I knew what that meant, and I wished I'd prepared myself better. I hadn't yet filled my prescription for Zofran for nausea.

Stupid on my part!

The day lasted so long I had just wanted to go home, not make yet another stop and wait for who knows how long until the pharmacist filled the prescription. Everyone told me precautions had been taken to prevent nausea, and indeed I didn't feel sick when we got home. I should have known better. I'd been overconfident. My first mistake. There would be more.

An almost-full moon shined through the twin skylights in our bathroom, making it unnecessary to turn on a light. Supporting myself with shaking arms, one on either side of the bathroom sink, I peered at my face in the mirror. I looked worn and unhappy, but otherwise like me. I dragged myself to our guest room, the same room that had been my mother's.

I was shivering, my shoulders and legs shaking. I couldn't get warm. In the guest room closet I found an afghan I had crocheted years ago and wrapped it around myself. I then sat up in an upholstered chair next to a window, propping my feet on the nearby bed. My past experience with nausea had taught me that sitting upright for a few hours might allow me to get through the spell without vomiting.

My head pounded. I closed my eyes. I ached all over. I opened my mouth and took slow breaths to control my queasiness. I had an urge to swallow, but every time I did, I had pain from Tuesday's surgery. Sleep, of course, was out of the question.

I didn't see any point in waking Chris up. To hold my hand again? He'd been good about that, but I didn't need to wake him up just to watch me feel sick. Even after all the years of intimate married life, some things remained too personal to share, and vomiting was one of them. I didn't want my husband's image of me to be of greenish fluid pouring out of my mouth.

As I sat in that chair in the dark room, fighting against vomiting, exhausted but awake, I gave in to every worry I'd tried to stifle in the past month.

I tried to convince myself that I wasn't in such a bad spot. My cancer was potentially curable. I had great doctors and a caring and supportive family and friends. I had been fortunate enough to be given a treatment option that avoided extensive and risky surgery, wide radiation, and a harsh chemotherapy agent that would have made my side effects much worse. Until then I had no first-hand knowledge of those side effects. However, sitting upright in a chair in the middle of the night, I was filled with dread.

It could be much worse! I just have to show up, obey my doctors, and push myself through the next few months. I can do this!

But what am I in for? Can I do this?

Sometimes my knowledge of anatomy and medicine was a curse more than a benefit because it brought to mind everything that could go wrong. This was one of those times when ignorance would have been bliss. I began ticking off the vulnerable structures in my mouth and neck Dr. Layan had mentioned on the day of my radiation simulation.

During my career I had spent a few years as an x-ray technician, and I knew that a beam of radiation passes through tissue in a straight line. Radiation would kill not just my tumor but also much of what it passed through. Also, some radiation is absorbed by the tissue through which it travels and can then spread from that central point to damage nearby tissues and organs.

Clearly, much more tissue was involved than the tumor in my tongue. We take simple, automatic functions, like swallowing, for granted. Like everyone else, I never thought of the structures in my body individually before their existence was jeopardized. They just worked. Until they didn't.

So much went on in an area only five inches wide, five inches deep, and five inches tall. How many structures would be affected? I was unlikely to come out of this with no damage at all.

My teeth were likely to weaken and decay. How many might I lose?

Robbie, the radiation oncology nurse, told me the lining of my mouth and my gums would get inflamed and produce a slimy, foul-tasting coating. That sounded unpleasant, but there were other things that worried me more.

Such as my tongue, the culprit in this whole awful deal. Would I lose part of it? Would I still be able to talk and to work food around in my mouth? My taste buds were on my tongue, too. I had been told I was likely to lose most of my sense of taste. Some of my sense of taste should return, but how much was unknown. Would I ever enjoy food again? Or regain my appetite?

Salivary glands produced secretions that kept the lining of my mouth healthy and moist. Saliva mixed with food so it could be worked into a mass I could swallow. Absence of saliva would be unpleasant and would also allow unhealthy bacteria to grow and make me sick. Saliva also contains enzymes that help reduce tooth decay. Another reason my teeth would be at risk for years.

Would I be able to swallow at all? Would I need a feeding tube, like my mother had, and have to be fed through a hole in my side? The idea terrified me.

Some of the bone in my face, especially in my jaw, could die from radiation. What would my life be like if I lost part of my jaw, and how disfigured might I be?

My tongue is surrounded by vital organs: my ears, my nose, and the eustachian tube that controls pressures between these organs, like when your ears pop in an airplane. My ears, nose, and eustachian tube would all be in or near the path of radiation. Not only my hearing, but my sense of balance could be affected. Even before I had cancer I suffered from periodic lightheadedness and occasional vertigo. Would I still be able to control that? And the base of my brain sat right on top of it all and would receive some radiation as well.

My brain! My blood supply, nerves! The muscles in my face! Stop!

A new wave of nausea rose in my throat, and suddenly I was hot instead of cold. I threw off the afghan and began to breathe deeply and rhythmically through my open mouth, counting each breath. I'd try to get to one hundred before I gave in and rushed to the bathroom. Slowly the nausea faded again, and I spent a few moments gazing out the bedroom window as the bright moonlight on the cold, cloudless night threw ominous shadows across my front lawn and down the street. The world, it seemed, had no concern for my misery, but reflected my mood.

I had controlled the moment of panic, but the thoughts, like the ominous shadows on my lawn, returned, so I forced myself to consider my situation logically. Cold again, I covered myself with the afghan once more and then put my fingers against the angles of my jaw. I imagined the path of radiation traveling from the point of one jaw to the other, targeting areas within a few inches of that line.

I gently pressed on my neck, exploring the area where the first swollen gland was found. There was nothing unusual to be felt there now. I ran my fingers up and down, exploring the tense muscles at the sides and back of my neck, which held my head up. My doctors said cancer had spread to some of those muscles. I paused over the pulse in my carotid artery, beating steadily but hard due to my anxiety. Other major arteries and veins, those that supplied the brain, ran through my neck. So did nerves that controlled sensation and movement, the bone in my spine, and the spinal cord that carried instructions between my brain and the rest of my body. Lymph nodes and lymphatic ducts ran along my jaw, in my neck, and carried lymphatic fluid to other parts of my body. There was already cancer in some of those too.

I poked a finger around my voice box, immediately below my jaw. I couldn't feel anything unusual, no tenderness or lump...now. But my voice box would obviously receive some radiation. How would that affect my voice? Would I still be able to sing? I couldn't see myself sitting in the audience instead of experiencing the joy of performing. Would my epiglottis continue to function and prevent me from aspirating food into my lungs when I swallowed? That reminded me of the feeding tube again.

Then I remembered that thyroid and parathyroid glands surround my larynx. They produce hormones that control metabolism, how my body uses energy and calcium.

Would my throat or airway swell to the point that I wouldn't be able to breathe? Would I need a tracheostomy?

How is it ever going to be possible to protect and preserve everything from radiation?

Let alone chemotherapy. Correction, monoclonal antibodies. Chemo could affect other parts of my body than my neck. What was going to happen there? I understood my therapy would be easier, but easier compared to what?

I supposed I had to entertain these thoughts somewhere along the line. Entertain. Not the best word to use...

All my years working in the medical field, I thought my knowledge gave me an advantage. I remembered a wise man I respected saying that a little knowledge was dangerous. How much of an advantage did my experience actually give me? Would I be better off as an average patient?

I must go through this to kill the cancer. But how much of me will remain?

Again, I could do nothing other than show up, follow directions, trust my medical team to do what they do, and pray that most of my function would return.

After two hours of torturing myself with thoughts like these, terrified but exhausted, I was finally able to return to bed and fall asleep.

In the morning my nausea was still present. I sent Chris out to get my prescription for Zofran filled and began taking it, but I stayed in bed most of that day.

Getting up midmorning to use the bathroom, I stared at my worn face in the mirror again and ran my fingers through my uncombed hair. I felt something behind my left ear. I had forgotten the scopolamine patch that the anesthetist placed when I had my biopsy. I should have removed it the following day but had forgotten. I wondered why it hadn't prevented the nausea I was still having.

I picked up my phone and looked up the drug. I read that one of the lesser side effects of a patch that was intended to prevent nausea was, amazingly, nausea.

If anyone is going to get nausea instead of stop nausea, it will be me!

I peeled off the patch and went back to bed.

Bob called during his lunch.

"I'm sorry you're feeling bad, but this isn't entirely unusual, Mom. This won't last. Don't forget, you had a larger dose of Cetuximab this time. You should try to get out of bed. And eat something. Remember, you have to keep up your strength. That's not going to happen lying in bed and starving yourself. And drink plenty of water."

"Yes, Doctor Bob," I mumbled.

I did try. The Zofran did not stop the nausea, but it wasn't as bad. Or maybe taking off the patch helped. Gradually, the extreme weakness wore off. I couldn't eat, but I did drink my first bottle of Ensure, which had been given to me in oncology. By seven in the evening, I was able to sit up in a recliner and watch television with Chris for a couple of hours before going back to bed for the night.

The following day I ate small meals and took a short walk.

Three days after the first infusion, I had no headache, no nausea, only slight lightheadedness, more energy, and a little appetite started to return.

When I came downstairs that morning, Chris was standing at the kitchen sink, making coffee.

"So far this isn't too bad," I said. "I was only sick a couple of days. The next dose will be half. I think I can do this."

I watched Chris's face, hoping to see reassurance there. What I saw was more like relief. I realized he may have been more scared than I had been but hidden it from me—sometimes it's even harder on the spouse. The thought brought tears to my eyes.

Misunderstanding my tears, Chris dried his hands and hugged me. "We're going to do this," he said.

Later that afternoon, I went into the closet where I had stored my yarn, patterns, and knitting and crochet materials. I hadn't done much needlecraft since I started writing novels, but I was sure what I needed would be on hand. I was a sucker for sales and had bought way too much yarn during the many years I spent more time crafting hats, scarves, afghans, sweaters, and the like.

As I expected, I found full skeins of a soft, baby-blue yarn and a pattern for a newborn cap. Dr. Fidler's baby boy would have a cap to come home from the hospital.

CHAPTER 21
Second Infusion and Postoperative Visit
Thursday, January 11, 2018

"I wish we could have been more involved. We kept checking on you and you were doing fine. Chris was very helpful. It was more of a burden on him than any of us." - Dolly, daughter-in-law

Thursday, January 11, a week after my first infusion, was an even longer day than the day I had the first chemo.

I arrived at the cancer center at 9:30 that morning. That time an assistant took me to a laboratory in the same suite, where a phlebotomist took my blood. Then she moved me to an examination room and an oncology nurse checked my vital signs. I saw Mary, the nurse practitioner, Mandy, the study coordinator, and then Dr. Fidler.

"How did you do after your first infusion?" Dr. Fidler asked.

"I was pretty sick the first night—nausea, headache, extreme weakness, dizziness. Zofran didn't stop my nausea completely but helped."

"That's not unusual after a first dose," she said. "Today you're getting a regular dose, not double, and that shouldn't be as bad. Due to your nausea, though, I'll add another premedication. That should take care of the problem." She searched my eyes. "We don't want you to be sick."

Chris and I exchanged glances. One of my worst fears was realized with the first infusion and I was dreading a repeat of that experience today. I still doubted my nausea could be eliminated but was pleased that she addressed the issue without my having to beg.

"Have you been eating? Exercising? Active during the day?"

"I don't have much appetite, but I'm trying. I started counting calories, and I'm getting about 1200 most days. I try to walk on an indoor track every day for twenty or thirty minutes. I'm not feeling as weak, and the pain in my throat is getting better."

"That's good. Are you sleeping okay?"

"Yes, surprisingly. I usually have a hard time sleeping when I'm stressed."

"Your body is not only fighting your cancer, but the chemo is taking some of your energy too. You'll need more rest, but you should engage in as much of your normal activity as possible without overdoing it. Try not to focus too much on your disease."

As if I can do that when my days are all planned around fighting cancer!

Chris and I walked down to the infusion waiting room. The receptionist looked up. "They're ready for you. You can go right in."

This time the infusion nurse took us to a pod to the left of the nurses' desk near a wall of windows.

Like the previous week, a nurse placed an IV in my hand, verified my identity, and scanned my bracelet and all vials of medication.

"I understand you were sick after your first infusion. Sometimes the first one is tough. From now on we're adding Axoli to your premedication injection. That should take care of it."

I was skeptical that anything would prevent my nausea. However, I knew that, even if I did get sick, it would be unpleasant but not devastating. I could handle it. The first infusion itself went smoothly without problems or discomfort, so I felt confident that this time the experience would go equally well.

I had remembered to empty my bladder before entering the room, and we had brought hard-boiled eggs and some crackers and cheese. Chris and I snacked, and then I pulled out my Kindle and read while Chris looked at magazines.

All went well and, like the previous week, I felt a little tired, which could have been because I'd been sitting for almost three hours. I wasn't sick, the experience seemed easy, and I was relieved.

By 12:30 we were on our way to our next appointment.

On Thursdays Dr. Thomas had appointments at Rush Oak Park Hospital instead of the main downtown Rush Medical Center campus. The drive took about a half hour. He wanted to see me to be sure there were no problems after last week's biopsy and to answer any remaining questions I might have. Dr. Thomas was his usual cheerful self.

Surgeons have a reputation for advising surgery, which is their expertise, over other methods of treatment. Despite all the opinions that the option I chose was effective, I wanted his reassurance again that I had made the right decision.

"Umm...I'm not sure how to ask this...are you sure what we're doing will work? That I shouldn't have had surgery instead?" I said.

He sat on a stool in front of the exam table and took both my hands in his. "I'm good at what I do. But in this case surgery wouldn't be what's best for you," he said. "Cutting out cancer is the surest, but not always the best, option. Not all tongue cancers receive radiation the same way, depending on the pathology of the tumor, its size and location, how close it is to other structures, whether it's spread—where, and how much—and the patient's general health. Some people need surgery, some need chemotherapy, some need radiation, and some need a combination of these therapies."

He paused for a moment to be sure I'd understood.

"We recommended your option because your cancer has spread to your neck. Surgery would be extensive and carry a risk for functional and cosmetic damage, such as loss of your voice box or mandible. On the plus side, your cancer hasn't spread anywhere else. The combination of radiation and chemotherapy, in the oncology team's opinion, will be safe, effective, and avoid the risks of surgery."

As he talked, I remembered a woman I met who had been disfigured by facial surgery after an auto accident many years ago. The left side of her face was caved in where her jaw should be, and she could barely close her mouth. Her nose was pushed upward, her two large nostrils apparent. Her face reminded me of Edvard Munch's painting, *The Scream*. The injuries left her with garbled speech and difficulty eating. Would surgery leave me like that? I felt suddenly cold and a little disoriented.

"But...how do we know this treatment will be enough?" My voice was almost a whisper.

"Your radiation will be targeted to areas we know are diseased and those areas where your cancer is most likely to spread, using higher doses for cancerous areas and lower doses to remaining areas. These days we know a lot about how squamous cell tumors at the base of the tongue spread, and those areas receive attention."

"So, surgery wouldn't be safer for me?" I'd been through these concerns with other doctors before I agreed to the trial, but Dr. Thomas had been my doctor for years and had never given me bad advice. I wanted to hear what he had to say.

"Radiation kills normal cells along with the cancer, but only those in the field of radiation. It causes less damage than surgery. If any cancer remains after treatment, we could operate at that time. But in that case surgery would involve only the remaining disease, less extensive.

"The object, of course, is to kill all existing cancer cells while harming as little as possible of your normal, healthy cells. Having chemotherapy at the same time will stop the growth of cancer cells in other parts of your body and prevent their spread."

Hearing these facts detailed so clearly made me realize I had narrowly escaped something dreadful. I was optimistic.

CHAPTER 22
First Radiation Therapy Treatment
Thursday, January 11, 2018 – Late Afternoon

"I was surprised to hear you had to wear a mask, how they aimed the treatment, and the details of how modern medicine worked. I read a book and watched a TV show to try to get an idea of what it was like for you."
- Clare, daughter-in-law

Chris and I were in a good mood as we left Dr. Thomas's office to drive back to Rush Medical Center and radiation oncology. During the ride my anxiety started to build once again. I imagined myself fixed to the table by my mask, unable to move, while radiation was zapped at me.

Having studied almost forty years ago to be an x-ray technician, I had a good grasp of how things worked. But using radiation diagnostically as I did was not the same as using it to destroy tumors. I didn't expect to feel anything during the treatment, but I'd never actually had radiation. What if something did happen? The intent was to kill cells in my body, after all. Once treatment began, there would be no turning back from that point on—unless I gave up or it failed, neither of which I wanted to think about. I had no idea how my body would react. Would I be able to withstand what was to come?

Because it was late in the day by the time we arrived, almost four in the afternoon, I was relieved to find there were parking spaces available in the area we were told we could park free. There appeared to be only about ten spaces, though. I wondered how easy it would be to find one earlier in the day when it was busier. Hospital parking could be a challenge.

"Our parking pass actually worked," I told Chris. "I was afraid we'd have to drive over to the regular lot and walk back."

When we entered through the automatic doors into the reception area, Sheryl, the receptionist, looked up. "Hi Pat. How are you doing today?" She smiled kindly. "Don't look so worried. We're going to take good care of you here."

I smiled back, impressed that she knew my name without my needing to tell her. I was also impressed that she noticed my apprehension and tried to reassure me.

When I was responsible for a medical practice at Rush, I had always stressed to my staff that little courtesies like using names, a smile, and a friendly face meant a lot to patients. I would have hired this lady in a minute.

The male receptionist gave me a smile and a nod. "You're a little early, but that's good this late in the day. Have a seat and you'll be called soon."

After ten minutes, I heard over the loudspeaker, "Mrs. Camalliere, we're ready for you."

I remembered the routine from last week: go through the double doors and enter the department; a few doors down on the right was the changing room; take off everything above my waist and put on a gown; sit down and wait for my therapist to come for me. This time I was proactive, stepped into the bathroom in the changing area, and emptied my bladder before I returned to the changing room to wait for someone to come for me.

Paul arrived shortly and engaged me in small talk as we walked together down the hall. He walked next to me, matching his pace to mine, not ahead and expecting me to follow. Little things like that were comforting.

When I entered the treatment room, at first I thought someone was already on the table. Someone, probably Vani, had placed my mask where my head and shoulders would soon be. I smiled, feeling that my therapists were well prepared, that they welcomed and cared for me.

Vani entered the room, picked up the mask, and helped me onto the table.

"It is always cold in this room for the therapy unit to work properly," she said in her quiet but clipped tones. "If you wear a tank top and do not wear your bra the next time you come, you do not need to change. You can come right to this room, and you will be warmer too."

I smiled at her, appreciating the thoughtfulness.

"Do you have any questions before we start?" Paul asked. He stood in front of me with his hands in the pockets of his white lab coat.

"Why did I have to wait a week after I came in for my mask?" I asked. I knew at least part of the answer, but I was always curious about what happened behind the scenes. Since I was going to be seeing these people Monday through Friday for thirty-five days, I wanted to establish a rapport, and I also wanted them to know I was more familiar with medical terms and procedures than the average patient. In other words, I hope they got the "don't talk down to me" message.

Paul didn't withhold the medical jargon. Perhaps he knew my background.

"We needed the week to work out your treatment plan. Dr. Layan, along with our radiation dosimetrists and physicists, carried out a careful, slide-by-slide delineation process of your CT scan, defined your treatment field, and pinpointed exactly where the radiation beam will be aimed.

"They mark each critical structure in the field, the areas that need to be treated, and the optimal dose distribution for each treatment area. These criteria are calculated over a thirty-five-dose plan by our dosimetrists. Then our physicists, who are responsible for quality assurance, check the calculations.

"The last step is after all three—the dosimetrists, the physicists, and Dr. Layan—agree. Then they run the plan on a phantom patient on this same machine."

The elaborate and painstaking process was even more technical than I expected. If I couldn't follow every detail, I got the gist of what he said, which was not only impressive but reassuring. I hoped my expression convinced Paul that I wasn't completely baffled by his explanation, although I was bluffing a bit.

Paul asked me to lie on the table and positioned me carefully. "This machine is called a TomoTherapy unit. It will deliver many small beams of radiation at your tumor from different angles to get the best dose distribution, as defined in your plan.

"Radiation does not kill cancer cells immediately, but they will continue to die over the course of the treatment, and even for weeks or longer *after* your therapy is finished. During the course of the treatment your body needs to rest and catch up. That's why you skip Saturday and Sunday."

I giggled. "I thought that was because you didn't want to work on weekends."

He laughed with me. "It's a mutual benefit."

Vani covered me with a blanket taken from the warmer. I had been shaking since I entered the room. How much of this was from nerves and how much from the temperature in the room I wasn't sure, but the blanket was a blessing.

"Ready?" she asked.

When I nodded, Paul and Vani, one on each side of the table, placed my mask over my face and shoulders and fastened it to the table. It was very tight. I couldn't fully open my eyes, but I could see a little above and to the sides through the mesh. The plastic pressed against my nose, but I could breathe normally. I could barely wiggle my lips, but they parted enough that my voice could be heard. My shoulders were tight against the table. My arms, however, were free. Vani clipped an oxygen monitor on one finger, and carefully covered my arms with the blanket. I welcomed the warmth.

Paul and Vani left the room, leaving me alone. I had been told I wouldn't feel anything during treatment, so I wasn't worried about that. I *was* worried that I wouldn't be able to hold still, even with the mask; about the eventual outcome of my therapy; and about side effects that would happen later. I told myself that I should just rest and let the therapists do the work. I had nothing to do for the half hour or so the entire process would take. I found myself feeling glad that I had free time to pursue my own thoughts, mostly curiosity about what was going to happen.

Some people complain of claustrophobia when being drawn into a therapy machine. I'd never been claustrophobic, but there I was, fastened to a table by my mask and unable to move while radiation was beamed into me. The situation certainly had a potential to give me that "let me out of here" fight-or-flight panic.

To prepare, I had studied some meditation techniques, but in the end I decided praying would work better. The repetition of saying memorized prayers is calming and slows my heart rate, like counting sheep. And prayer carries the further benefit of reassurance from heaven. That could never hurt. Conclusion: I would pray if I started to panic.

Despite the fact that I knew I was a control freak who didn't like to have anything taken out of my hands or to be confined in any way, now that I was actually in position, I found my mask to be oddly comforting, similar to how a baby must feel when swaddled. I could see enough of the room that being drawn into the donut was not alarming, and I had the reassurance of knowing the mask would help me keep motionless, making the radiation most effective.

Over a loudspeaker I heard: "We're going to start your CT now."

Soon I felt the table begin to move, and I was drawn into the "donut," or "bore." I was surrounded by the whiteness of the machine. Then there was a whirring noise, as if something was warming up, and then a loud clunk. I remembered what Paul had told me.

"The first thing we'll do is take a CT scan, so we have a record of today's exact position. Then we'll lay today's scan over the details of your planning CT, matching each area to be radiated to be sure that it gets the accurate dose for today. Think in 3-D. The scan takes multiple 'slices,' or images, and these have to be matched to multiple areas of delivery and the dosage planned for each."

Even with the mask in place, I was careful not to move. I had an urge to clear my throat, to swallow, and to wrinkle my nose and my lips. I'd been told that wouldn't affect the scan, but I wanted to be sure that I didn't screw anything up, and so I tried not to make any movements like that.

The equipment clicked and clunked and moved in little bursts, and after about three minutes, the table slid me out of the donut. I heard Paul again over the loudspeaker: "We've finished the scan. It will be a little while now until today's matching is done."

I was told to expect a pause while the therapists completed the matches. The actual delivery of the radiation, which would happen next, took about ten minutes. And so, I was left to my thoughts again. I could flex my muscles, move my hands, swallow, and wiggle. I realized, now that I could swallow and wiggle somewhat freely, I no longer had a desire to.

I heard Paul's voice again. "We're going to start delivering today's dose now."

The whirring began again, I was drawn into the bore again, and the sounds were unlike what I'd heard before. It sounded to me like continuous rattling that circled around the donut, around my head, neck, and shoulders. It made me wonder if the machine was broken. Was it supposed to make noises like that? Should I move my legs violently to catch the therapists' attention and have them stop the procedure, like they told me? Surely they'd notice if something was wrong. I kept expecting the unit, or the noise, to stop suddenly, but it didn't.

And then an amusing thought occurred to me. The rattling made an image appear in my mind, the image of a shaman or medicine man, like the one I wrote about in *The Mystery at Black Partridge Woods*. I envisioned a scantily clad man holding a rattle, ceremoniously conducting a healing ritual by dancing around me and the therapy machine. Instead of alarming, the sound became a friendly and familiar one, and I welcomed it.

The rattling, and the therapy, lasted about seven minutes. I didn't feel anything happening in my body. Sort of. Now and then I thought there could be a slight pressure in the area I knew was being treated. Toward the end of the delivery, I thought my throat could be a little warm. It was probably in my mind, which was on extreme alert for anything unusual.

And then it was over. We said goodbyes, I returned to the dressing room, changed back into my street clothes, and left the department with Chris. We walked out into the dark. I hoped that starting for home toward the end of rush hour would make the ride shorter than usual.

Another long day, but once again everything went smoothly. I didn't get sick from my chemo—so far—but the night was yet to come. I had spent the day racing from appointment to appointment, but I ran on time and had no bad experiences anywhere. I was calm, relieved, but proud of myself for staying upbeat.

I didn't have to pray, because of my unexpected company. After all, what could possibly go wrong with that little man waving his rattle and dancing around me?

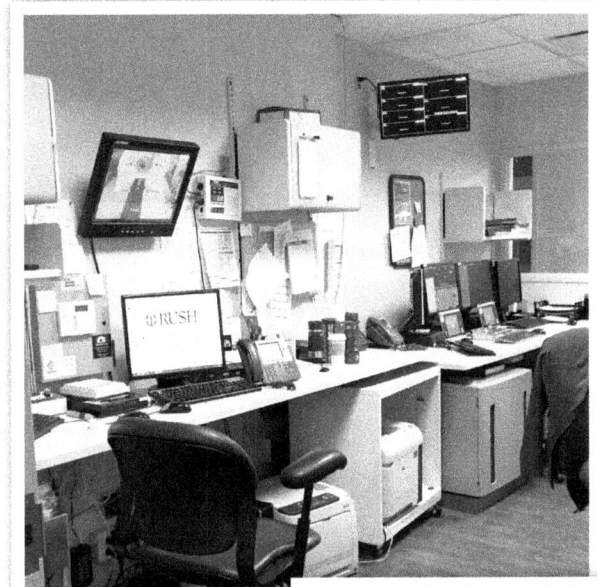

The radiation "control room."

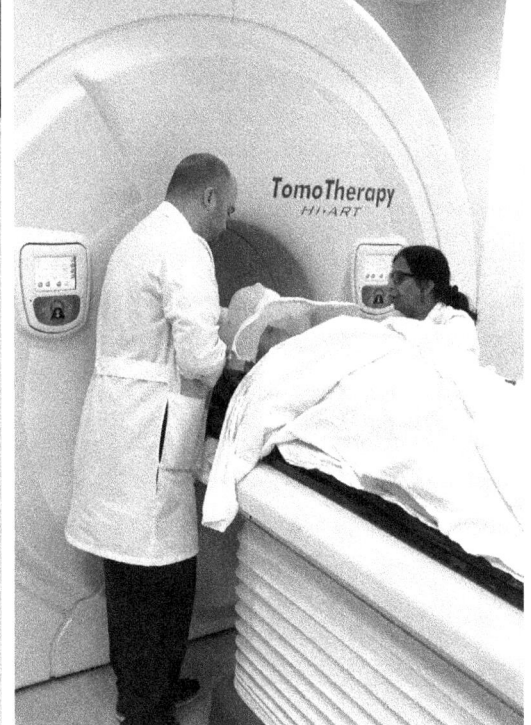

Paul and Vani attaching my mask in the TomoTherapy unit.

CHAPTER 23
Life Before Cancer: Single Parent, 1980-1990

The interests and goals Frank and I shared at the beginning of our marriage slowly changed. In the 1960s, more women were getting degrees, but most still married soon after finishing their education. We had followed the customary expectation. We married two months after I graduated and started a family right away.

Or perhaps we were too inexperienced and confused fondness with love. I wanted to go out and enjoy activities with my family; he wanted to stay home and save money. He didn't understand things that were important to me, and I couldn't figure out what was important to him. Probably neither of us was right nor wrong, we just realized we saw things differently. Little by little, we grew further apart and divorced in 1980.

It had been years since Frank and I had been comfortable together, so living in the same house had been stressful. After the divorce, life was hard. John and Bob lived with me in the same home, and they continued to go to the same schools and see their friends. I still worked at the medical center, where I ran the practice for twenty-two years, twelve years as a single parent. My work was very demanding, but somehow, we got through those challenging teen years together. John and Bob both graduated high school and then entered college.

When John and Bob both finished college with degrees in engineering from the University of Illinois on the same day, proud Mom was there at the graduation. Soon John started working as an engineer at a nuclear power plant for what was then Commonwealth Edison, and then married Clare. Bob moved to Detroit to become an engineer for Ford Motor Company.

Because I had friends with sons who dragged their feet about getting jobs after college and lived with their parents for years, I had told John and Bob that they would be welcome to live with Chris and me for a year after graduation, but after that I would expect them to contribute to the household income. I said this with the expectation that after college they would come back to me, and I would have them again for a little while.

I don't know whether it was because of my words on the matter, or just coincidental, but after college Bob moved immediately to the job waiting for him in Detroit, and John was with me only two weeks before starting work in Zion, Illinois.

I was proud. But I was sad. I had looked forward to that time with them again. I felt cheated when they moved away so soon.

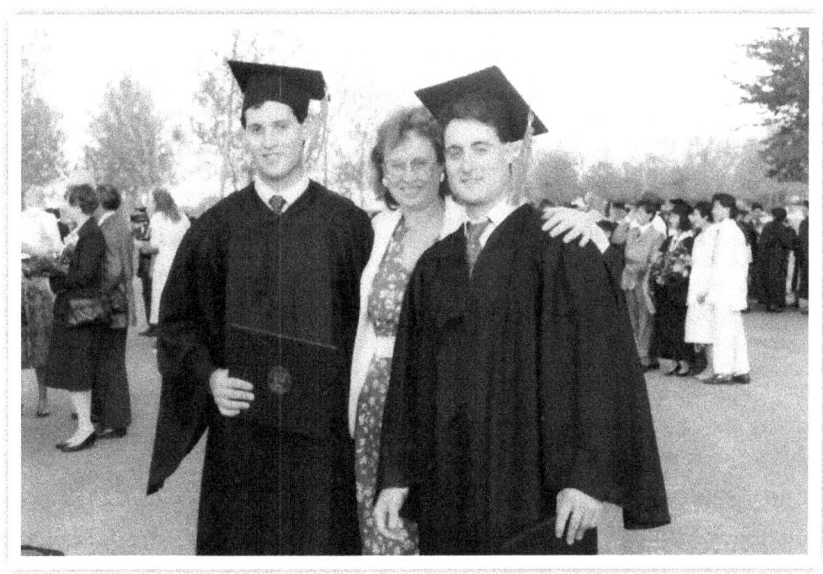

Me with John and Bob, University of Illinois graduation.

CHAPTER 24
Chemotherapy

"You do your best, but it is a nasty disease that does whatever it wants. You can also enter with one thing and end up with something different that pops up later." - Dolly, daughter-in-law

Thankfully, I slept through the night after my second infusion and felt only mild nausea when I awoke. The second delivery of radiation the next day on Friday, January 12, went as smoothly as the first, and then I had the weekend with no appointments. Things were going better than I expected. I had no side effects and began to relax about the entire process. I believed, as my doctors had predicted, everything would go well.

The PET scan I had before treatment began showed that my cancer had not spread past my neck. The scan looked at other areas where this type of cancer usually did or could spread, such as the lungs. I didn't show cancer in those areas, only those we already knew about in my tongue and neck.

But was there microscopic spread that didn't show on the scan? This wasn't likely, but it wasn't impossible. With cancer, the last thing I wanted to do was take a chance or ignore something until it was too late. I imagined a tiny little bad guy invading my bloodstream. He wore a yellow leather crossbody pouch, an evil version of Johnny Appleseed, circling my body, scattering cancer seeds instead of apple seeds. I wanted that little demon gone!

That was why I was getting Cetuximab: to improve the effectiveness of radiation therapy and increase the likelihood of a cure. It covered the parts of my body that were not undergoing radiation.

I had been told that a simple explanation of how a monoclonal antibody kills cancer is that it works with the body's own immune system. The not-so-simple explanation is that it blocks the function of a protein called EGFR, or epidermal growth factor receptor, which causes cells to grow and divide. Cetuximab, an EGFR inhibitor, binds with and "tags" cancer cells so they will not grow and allows the body's immune system to seek out and kill them.

The word "kill" stuck in my mind. It was a word I didn't use much before it gained a more immediate importance in my life. The word was still uncomfortable to me as I grappled with the question of whether, with the help of modern medicine, we would kill my cancer, or if it would kill me. This was a very real battle I was engaged in, a battle that only one of us could win—no ties allowed here. But my decisions were made; the fight had begun. I didn't want to focus on death, but on doing whatever I could to get rid of the demons in my body.

In my case, I saw man and science working hand in hand with God—the combination of Cetuximab and my own body's defenses. Medical science finds a way to trigger God's handiwork to do the job, and we marvel at the result.

I had radiation Monday through Friday, and every Thursday for eight weeks I also had a "chemo day." On chemo day I went back and forth between two buildings in the Rush Medical Center complex, with wait times between appointments. It took all day.

Each chemo day I packed a little striped bag with a silver insulated lining. It contained everything I needed, including comfort items and things to keep me busy during waiting periods. The bag came from an organization on Facebook, #BetterEveryDay. A friend had enrolled me when she found out I had cancer, and I received a welcome package that included the bag. Throughout the next few months, I received occasional messages of encouragement both on Facebook and in the mail. Little gifts also arrived, such as a packet of handmade get-well cards from schoolchildren.

In that bag I packed lunch and a snack, a spoon, containers of mouth rinse, hand sanitizer, and the medications I needed to take during the day.

Nurses would bring me a warm blanket, but I also brought a sweater and a throw for longer waiting periods. I dressed in comfortable clothes and shoes, elastic-waisted knit pants and loose tops. I brought my Kindle and my iPhone, and Chris brought a magazine.

Chris drove me to Rush every day and accompanied me to my appointments. On chemo day we usually left the house about nine in the morning for a one-hour trip—avoiding rush hour traffic—and were on our way home by four in the afternoon. I got some things done in the car while Chris drove, like therapy exercises.

We parked in the radiation oncology lot adjacent to the main hospital building, using our free pass, and walked first to the cancer center in the Professional Building. A phlebotomist drew my blood, and then I was taken to an exam room, where I saw Mary, my nurse practitioner, followed by Mandy, my clinical study coordinator, and last Dr. Fidler. It was usually late morning before I saw everyone. My infusion wouldn't be calculated and prepared by the pharmacy until afternoon.

My appointment in radiation oncology was at one in the afternoon. If time allowed between appointments, I took my medications when due, applied skin lotions, used the restroom, or performed routines on my daily care list. Usually, the wait time was short, but sometimes it wasn't.

On the far side of the oncology waiting room was a little lunchroom with two round tables and chairs, a sink, a microwave, a single-cup coffeemaker, and a water dispenser. If there was time, Chris and I got something to drink and I ate the lunch I packed. I usually wasn't hungry, but I tried to eat something as I'd been told. To keep up my strength. For the fight. For killing my cancer. For stopping the little Johnny Appleseed bad guy from seeding cancer all over my body.

During those waits I read, checked emails, or played with my phone. Chris was patient, which I know was difficult for him. He read a magazine or dozed. Unlike me, he can sleep upright, and anywhere.

Then it was a ten-minute walk from the Cancer Center to the Radiation Oncology Department. I was glad we had to walk because, even if I was tired, it forced me to get some needed exercise. On days when I had time and energy, there were plenty of public places to walk in the Medical Center, and Chris and I would walk for thirty minutes.

After radiation therapy, we returned to Oncology for my infusion. By then it was mid-afternoon. There were usually three infusion nurses in the unit. I got to know them, and we chatted. One was a short, perky, thirtyish woman who worked for me years ago at University Surgeons. We shared a laugh over some memories of those days and caught up on our lives. The atmosphere in the infusion room was light, personal, and positive. The room was quiet and peaceful. I felt like I was among friends.

Nausea is not a common side effect of Cetuximab, but my first infusion *proved* that nausea *was* a problem for *me*. The addition of Aloxi made me more comfortable, but because nausea would prevent me from eating and good nutrition was vital to the success of my therapy, significant nausea would determine whether I would need to have a feeding tube placed.

After I arrived in my pod, my medications and other materials were assembled on a cart next to my recliner, and all information verified by scanners and computers as before. During my second infusion, the IV insertion didn't go so well. The nurse inserted the line into my hand like she did the first time, but before she finished hooking me up, the vein "blew" and began to leak blood under my skin. She withdrew the line without difficulty, but then she had trouble finding another vein to use. After a number of attempts, she successfully inserted the line into a vein above my wrist. This was not as comfortable as the first time because of bones just under the skin, but it was tolerable. Finally the line worked well, and the premedications were injected through the line. This was the only time there was a problem inserting the IV.

After the line was placed and the premedications given, I waited a half hour. During that time, the pharmacy delivered a small bag of clear fluid that contained my infusion. The bag and my wristband were scanned again, my nurse repeated my name, read the label on the bag, hung the bag, and set a program on the pump. A second nurse confirmed the information in the computer, verified the settings on the pump, and recorded the details of the infusion.

Yes, it's me. Yes, it's the right medicine. Yes, the pump is set right. Yes, it's all captured in the computer. Check and double-check. The bag was attached to the pump and the pump to my IV, and Cetuximab started to drip slowly into me. I didn't feel anything during the infusion, which took a bit over an hour.

Although my Kindle was within reach, I usually found I had little desire to read during the infusion. I tried a few times, but I couldn't detach myself enough from what was happening to focus on what I was reading. Instead, I ate a snack, checked my phone, or dozed. Fortunately, bathroom visits turned out not to be as worrisome as I feared, since I was literally being pumped full of fluids. The infusion pump ran on a battery, and once my nurse unplugged me from the wall, I could roll the cart and pump to a nearby restroom without assistance—although it was a little tricky.

The time usually passed quickly. I was tired by the time the nurse disconnected the pump and removed my catheter. Chris and I were free then, but it was late in the afternoon or early evening, and we always fought rush hour traffic. Unless something unusual happened, Chris and I didn't talk much in the car, only about things we saw during the ride. The premedications in the infusion had a calming effect on me, I was too tired, and we'd both experienced the same thing anyway.

We got home late. I would try to eat something, see if there were any phone calls to be answered, or deal with important mail. I would update my medical diary, check to be sure I finished everything on my medical to-do list. Then I'd crash in front of the television. Generally, I'd go up to bed before long.

Except for my first double-dose, I never felt weak or ill after an infusion. The Decadron I got before my infusions took two days to wear off, so instead I felt even better than usual for the first day or two after chemotherapy. Not only was I free of nausea, but I had a little energy boost that carried me through the days that often made other patients sick.

I began developing routines. At this early point I had very few side effects.

But I wondered how long treatment would continue to progress so well.

CHAPTER 25
Life Before Cancer: Chris and I Marry, 1991

Chris Camalliere was a salesman who came to my office monthly to talk about orders or problems we had with his company. We got to know each other and discovered we had both divorced during the same year. Over several years, this gave us common ground to talk about. We became casual friends. At lunch or after work we had lively discussions. I found it refreshing to be able to share my thoughts, problems, and plans with a man instead of my girlfriends.

Chris described himself as "medium everything." Medium height and weight, medium attractive, medium clothes sizes. As we became comfortable with each other, I realized that medium everything suited me just fine.

Both alone, we started seeing each other for dinner and then on weekends. At first, we talked about the things we were experiencing in our personal lives, but I began to notice little comforting things about Chris. Things like how we both bumped into each other accidentally when we walked, how we often had the same thought and caught each other's eye with no need for words, how he pitched in to help without waiting for me to ask. How he laughed off little problems and accepted bigger problems with determination. Or the sensation of his full palm against my back, not just an arm or a part of his hand. Or how he wrote down little messages when he had kind thoughts and left them for me without a spoken word. An attraction grew, and Chris and I married in 1991.

At our wedding, John gave me away, and Bob was the best man. Among the hundred friends and relatives present at our wedding was Bill, well-recovered from his lung surgery at Mayo.

A treasured memory of that day was how Bob ended his poignant "best man" speech.

"And now I'll ask the question that I'm sure is on everyone's mind: What took you guys so long?"

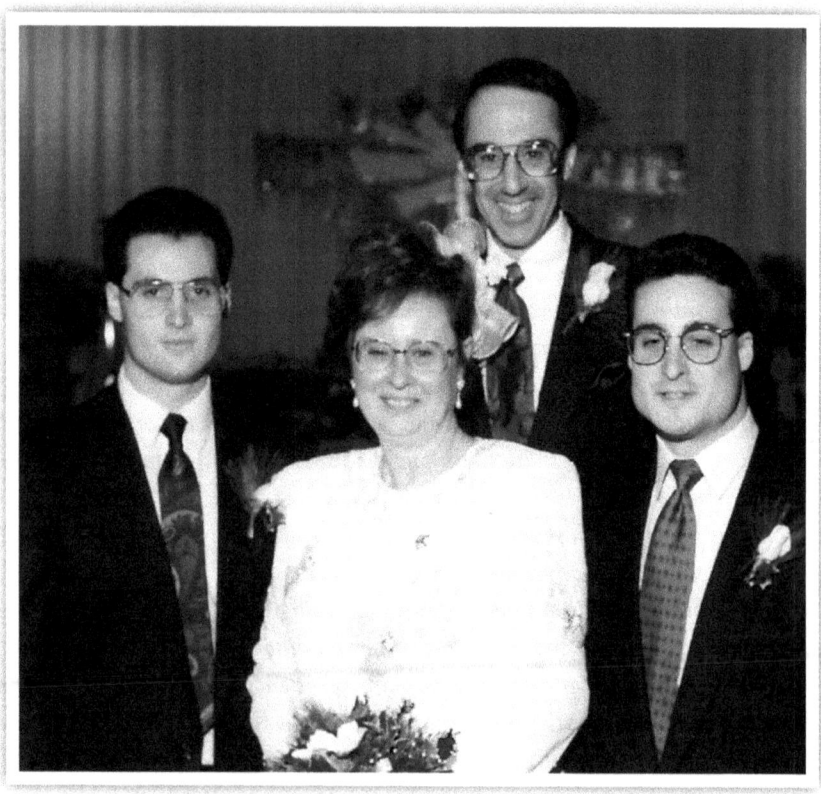

Wedding Photo: Me and Chris, John, and Bob

CHAPTER 26
A Day in the Life of a Cancer Patient

"I had to get up early, to the hospital back and forth every day, but it had to be and no big thing. But it took over everything. It was a daily thing."
- Chris, husband

"You figured out a lot of things every time we talked: what to eat, how to eat, what clothes to wear. Sometimes it's better to do your own things so long as you're not doing anything crazy. Too many opinions or options don't always help but just make more confusion." - Dolly, daughter-in-law

My life was going to be very different for a few months. I figured the sooner I accepted that and took steps to accommodate the changes, the better off I'd be. Being a head and neck cancer patient is a full-time job. I don't know how anyone can continue to work and fit in all that needs to be done, but apparently some do, and I admire them.

At the beginning of treatment, the biggest problems I had were worrying about what was going to happen and whether or not the treatment would do any good. Next the issue was adapting to new, time-consuming routines. Soon I found that my entire day was taken up with taking care of myself.

I remembered when I had cared for my mother. She saw therapists and nurses in our home every day, and had to do a variety of physical therapy, occupational therapy, and speech therapy exercises. She also had to take care of her feeding tube and take medications.

I can see her sitting in her customary place at our kitchen table, her back to the wall of windows that provided natural daylight and allowed her to read the newspaper and watch what was going on during the day. She had just finished her speech exercises and looked up to me, on her face an expression of disgust.

"Staying alive is a lot of work!" she complained.

I laughed at the time but didn't fully realize what she was feeling. After a couple of weeks of cancer treatment, I understood completely. I had no time for anything except staying alive.

"Surely you exaggerate," one might be inclined to say. I don't exaggerate.

The day of my first radiation treatment, Robbie, my nurse, told me I could make the next few months easier if I did certain things.

"Start now. Prevention is the key to success."

I agreed enthusiastically, anxious to make my journey easier. "Tell me what I have to do. I'll make it happen."

Once I committed to do my best, I quickly found there was a whole lot more to do than I expected. Most of it wasn't easy either. I had to fit a lot more routines into my day, and I was forgetting to do certain things or running out of time to do them.

Why?

First, there are appointments every day, Monday through Friday.

I resolved to be proactive from the beginning and took measures to minimize the side effects I was told to expect. Then later, when the side effects developed, I'd be better off.

"Put this lotion on twice a day. It will help with rashes and radiation burns. But don't put it on two hours before you have radiation therapy, or your burns will be worse." *Sounds a bit contradictory, but simple enough.*

"Use this mouth rinse four times a day. Don't put anything in your mouth for thirty minutes or longer afterward." *Okay—that's two hours though.... Alright, so I can do other things during that time, but can't a person exaggerate a little?*

"Salt rinses will help. Follow this recipe, use it four to six times a day, and don't put anything in your mouth for a half hour after." *Including time to make the mixture.... Hmmm—this is adding up.*

"Eat six small meals instead of three large ones." *Prep time plus eating* time, thirty minutes for each meal—that's another three hours.

"Get out and walk if you can. Thirty minutes a day is ideal."

"Speech therapy exercises—do them three times a day. Each session will take fifteen minutes."

"Brush your teeth after every time you eat, and swish with Biotene rinse." *Biotene didn't help me much when I used it before, but I'll give it a try again.*

"Take these new medications. Some are once a day, some twice, some every six hours, some only when you need them. Some you take with meals; others need to be on an empty stomach."

Stop already!

On top of everything I had to do at home every day, there were appointments for radiation and infusions and with doctors and therapists. Three to four hours were taken up every Monday through Friday getting to and keeping appointments in Radiation Oncology, and one long entire day when radiation therapy and chemotherapy fell on the same day.

I would lay out what I would wear the next day before I went to bed. Then, in case I was rushed or didn't feel well in the morning, I could shower, brush my teeth, and style my hair and makeup without taking time to search my closet for suitable clothes.

There were medications and routines I was doing before I started cancer treatment. Had to keep those up too. I was taking prescriptions for hypertension, elevated cholesterol, and esophageal reflux. I did daily exercises to prevent episodes of vertigo. The thought of getting a relapse of vertigo on top of nausea and dizziness that might occur during my therapy was terrifying. I had to fit that in my schedule.

Some activities had to be done in a certain order or spaced appropriately. I couldn't do this until I did that first, and once I did that, I had to follow with something else. For instance, if I rinsed my mouth right after I ate, what about those pills that were due at that time? I'd have to wait another half hour. So, I'd better move the pills up, take them before the rinse or I'd end up taking them too late in the day.

Much of what I needed to do related to some other activity. I'd begin something, then find out it was in the wrong order, and it set me back. My schedule started at seven in the morning and wasn't finished until ten at night. By two in the afternoon, I'd realize I wasn't finished with the ten o'clock morning hour yet.

Living with such chaos, always worried that I was forgetting something important enough to save my life, stressed me to the point that I had trouble thinking straight. I had to find a way to do this better. After all, I had run thriving medical practices and managed teams of professionals. Certainly I had the skills to manage my way through a day of cancer treatment. I should be able to distinguish between being organized and over-thinking.

For me the solution was a written schedule and check-off list. I wrote down everything I had to do and how many times I had to do it, gave each item a line and a time, and printed out a spreadsheet with boxes to check off what I did and mark what I missed.

I learned to juggle things that could be done simultaneously. For instance, since I had to wait thirty minutes after some rinses, I filled that time with other activities that didn't involve putting things in my mouth, like taking a shower or riding in the car. I found that drive time was a good time to get two sessions of speech therapy done, one on the way to the hospital and one on the way home. Only one more session to fit in—yay!

I put "mouth" activities in a progressive order: take pills first if they could be taken with food, then eat, then brush, use mouth rinses last.

The overwhelming number of details was confusing at first, so I didn't even try to make my schedule a permanent thing. I knew I'd be changing my spreadsheet as my side effects changed, new things were added, or I found a better order. So I printed a week at a time, made notes as I went along, and the next week I reassessed and printed a new schedule incorporating additions and discoveries. This turned out to be a smart decision.

Here's what my spreadsheet looked like. Sorry—it's pretty sloppy. It's good for one person—me—and it's a constant work in progress. It has shortcuts only I understand. There are too many variables, and no schedule could fit every patient. Each person's treatment is different, and each patient reacts differently, has different concerns, different side effects, different personal schedules, etc. I can't tell what everyone experiences, only what I experienced and what I did.

STAYING ALIVE IS A LOT OF WORK: ME AND MY CANCER

		FEB							
Time		Su	M	Tu	W	Th	F	Sa	Su
		28	29	30	31	1	2	3	4
7:30	Omeprazole - wait 30 min after (twice a day)	✓	✓	✓	✓	✓	✓	✓	✓
7:30	wash face and hydrocortisone (twice a day)	✓	✓	✓	✓	✓	✓	✓	✓
8:30	Salt rinse #1 (3 times a day)	✓	✓	✓	✓	✓	✓	✓	✓
8:30	Breakfast	✓	✓	✓	✓	✓	✓	✓	✓
8:30	Minocycline (twice a day - full glass water)	✓	✓	✓	✓	✓	✓	✓	✓
9:00	MuGard #1 - wait 30 min after (4 times per day)	✓	✓	✓	✓	✓	✓	✓	✓
10:00	Shower	✓	✓	✓	✓	✓	✓	✓	✓
10:00	Amlodipine	✓	✓	✓	✓	✓	✓	✓	✓
10:00	aspirin	✓	✓	✓	✓	✓	✓	✓	✓
10:00	Vitamin D	✓	✓	✓	✓	✓	✓	✓	✓
10:00	fluticasone	✓	✓	✓	✓	✓	✓	✓	✓
10:00	Cold cream wash and regenerist	✓	✓	✓	✓	O	✓	✓	✓
10:00	brush teeth and Biotene	✓	✓	✓	✓	✓	✓	✓	✓
10:00	lubricant - rectal if nec & other body creams	✓	✓	✓	✓	✓	✓	✓	✓
10:00	dizzy exercises (twice a day)	✓	✓	✓	✓	✓	✓	✓	✓
10:00	Bandaids if needed	O	O	O	O	✓	✓	✓	✓
10:00	Swallow exercises #1 (three times a day) 15 min	✓	✓	✓	✓	✓	✓	O	✓
11:00	morning snack	✓	✓	✓	✓	✓	✓	✓	✓
12:00	MuGard #2 - wait 30 min after (4 times per day)	✓	✓	✓	✓	O	✓	✓	✓
1:00	Salt rinse #2 (3 times a day)	✓	✓	✓	✓	O	✓	✓	✓
1:00	Lunch	✓	✓	✓	✓	✓	✓	✓	✓
1:00	brush teeth ~~and fluoride (twice a day) wait 30 min~~ biotene	O	✓	O	O	O	✓	O	✓
1:00	radiation therapy	O	✓	✓	✓	✓	✓	O	O
1:00	chemotherapy	O	O	O	O	✓	O	O	O
1:00	Skin lotion neck (twice a day) #1	✓	✓	✓	✓	✓	✓	✓	✓
2:00	walk 20-30 minutes	✓	✓	O	O	O	✓	O	O
3:00	afternoon snack	O	✓	O	O	O	✓	O	O
3:00	Swallow exercises (three times a day) 15 min #2	✓	✓	✓	✓	✓	✓	O	✓
3:00	MuGard - wait 30 min after (4 times per day) #3	✓	✓	✓	O	✓	✓	✓	✓
6:00	Swallow exercises #3 (three times a day) 15 min	O	O	O	O	O	O	O	O
6:00	Salt rinse #3 (3 times a day)	✓	O	O	O	✓	✓	✓	✓
6:00	dinner	✓	✓	✓	✓	✓	✓	✓	✓
6:30	Minocycline (twice a day - full glass water)	✓	✓	✓	✓	✓	✓	✓	✓
6:30	Miralax	✓	✓	✓	✓	✓	✓	✓	✓
7:00	floss and waterpik, brush and Biotene	✓	✓	✓	✓	O	✓	✓	✓
7:00	wash face and hydrocortisone (twice a day)	✓	✓	✓	✓	✓	✓	✓	✓
7:00	dizzy exercises (twice a day)	✓	✓	✓	✓	✓	✓	✓	✓
7:30	MuGard - wait 30 min after (4 times per day)	✓	O	✓	✓	O	O	✓	✓
8:30	Omeprazole - wait 30 min after (twice a day)	✓	✓	✓	✓	✓	✓	✓	✓
9:00	evening snack	✓	O	O	O	O	O	✓	O
9:00	toprol	✓	✓	✓	✓	✓	✓	✓	✓
9:00	pravastatin		✓	✓	✓	✓	✓	✓	✓
10:00	vagifem MWF	O	✓	O	✓	O	✓	O	O
10:00	estrace MWF		✓	O	✓	O	✓	O	O
10:00	clobetasol S-S-Tu-Th	✓	O	✓	O	✓	O	✓	✓
10:00	Skin lotion neck (twice a day)	✓	✓	✓	✓	✓	✓	✓	✓
10:00	Thick face cream	✓	✓	✓	✓	✓	✓	✓	✓
10:00	fluoride wait 30 min	✓	O	O	✓	O	O	O	O

I attached my checklist to a clipboard and carried it from place to place during the day so I didn't forget to check things off when I did them. I used a checkmark if I completed the item, a zero if I didn't. It was never perfect. It was just as easy to forget I'd done something and do it again as it was to miss something.

I certainly didn't get anything like a hundred percent done every day. There are zeroes on my checklist, but that's okay, because everything I did helped. Each day was different with different challenges and surprises. I didn't punish myself if I missed, but I did the best I could, and it made a difference.

Not everyone will be convinced that a check-off list like mine is necessary, but I believe working a schedule out on paper is well worth the time and effort spent. Many people get through busy days with no need for written lists or set timers on their Apple watch. It's a different matter when you're trying to do it while worried, unwell, and when changes occur frequently throughout the course of treatment. Developing routines helps, but they will be constantly changing and difficult to keep sorted. I'm willing to bet most people will get confused or forget a good deal of what they should be doing as treatment progresses. Progress it will, so don't make therapy harder than it needs to be. The sooner a person becomes an active participant, the more likely he is to be more comfortable throughout. Tools like lists can help.

No matter what the course turns out to be, it's the vast number of little time-consuming details that often exhausts the cancer patient.

In addition to a checklist, I also kept a journal. Each day I put the date and day of the week on the top of a new page in a composition book. As the day progressed, I wrote down my diet, condition, and symptoms: how I felt, when I started something new, when a new symptom started, what I ate in some detail, a calorie count, etc.

Here's what a typical day in my journal looked like:

> January 12 - Friday
> Slept fairly well - awoke alert about 4AM, mild
> headache, very mild nausea, no other effects. Fell back
> to sleep about 5:30-7:30.
> 150 Breakfast: ½ serving oatmeal 35/1 tsp butter 30, ½ tsp sugar 15 + blueberries 40
> 200   wheat toast w/ PB
> 30   coffee w/ creamer
>   Tongue is black - blueberries? (Frozen blueberries)
>   Small, difficult BM.
> 250 Lunch - PBJ + Cheese on roll (250)
> 220 Snack - Ensure
> 550 Dinner: fish (100) Mac + cheese w/ tuna (200) ½ shake (250)
>   Radiation therapy #2 - no side effects
>   Walked 30 min at hospital
>   Felt ok most of the day, less so after 6 PM
>   some warmth across upper chest
> 175 Snack: crackers + cheese
>
> Total
> 1575

I started this journal because all my medical team stressed from the beginning that my eating habits would change significantly through the course of my treatment. My doctors would ask me if I was getting enough nutrition and how eating changes affected my life. Once side effects occurred, I could report when they started, how long they lasted, and how severe they were. Also, I had something I could refer to in order to give my medical team good answers. The journal was bare bones, but I could easily look up and answer questions.

The journal also gave me personal satisfaction. I could compare what I'd recorded day to day to see if I was on track with my goals and measure how well I was doing.

My third "tool" was a notepad to bring to appointments. Whether I was seeing one of my doctors, nurses, or therapists, there was always useful, sometimes critical, information and instructions. I have a pretty good memory, but despite that I'd walk out of the room with two or three key things on my mind and forget many others if I didn't take notes during my appointments.

As the first month came to an end, I found it more and more difficult to find time for a daily walk. It got harder to get through a day without a nap. I had no energy for any activity after dinner, and I often fell asleep early in front of the television. There was little time to do anything except listen to my body.

My life had become all about treating cancer and taking care of myself. I realized, no matter how hard I tried, I couldn't do everything I wanted to. I had to quit expecting too much of myself, to put the rest of my life on hold until this was over and I could get well again. Thank God I had prepared well before starting treatment, but I was still surprised at how all-consuming cancer had become.

I sometimes wished I had a secretary and someone to stand over me and crack the whip. Chris was a tremendous help but was too kind to push me. I felt I had to be in control of my day-to-day schedule.

It wasn't so much that I was miserable as it was that my life had been taken over by my disease. I was tired. I tried to hide my feelings from my family and friends, but I was irritable because I didn't like having my life interrupted. I was used to doing what I wanted to do and making my own schedule. The need to add so many things made me grumpy, but also proud of myself sometimes.

The decision to postpone everything else in my life until this was over was a hard one for me, but making that decision motivated me to get treatment done and get well again.

Until that day came, I took satisfaction in the sense of accomplishment I got every time I picked up my daily list and checked an item off as done.

CHAPTER 27

Life Before Cancer: New Job and Elder Care, 1992-1998

Soon after Chris and I married, the clinic where I had worked for so long in Worth, Illinois was purchased by a local hospital, leaving me without my job. I found a new position as Administrator of University Surgeons at Rush University Medical Center and started commuting to the Chicago Medical District from the house we'd bought in Crestwood, a suburb southwest of Chicago.

I considered myself fortunate to work for University Surgeons. It was a good fit. I had twenty-two years of experience working in a private surgical practice. University Surgeons had recently formed a private group at an institution where most practices were hospital-owned. The doctors had no practice administration experience.

The surgeons in "my" group—"my boys," as I called them—had world class reputations. Patients were referred from around the world and celebrities were common.

Friends asked how difficult it was to work with prestigious surgeons. I never found it to be a problem. Yes, surgeons do tend to have big egos. But it takes a big ego to spend your career taking people's lives in your hands. I, for one, wouldn't want a surgeon who didn't have a big ego.

The trick was to always treat doctors with the respect that they deserved anyway. And when you had to propose something you thought they would *disagree with, present the issue in a way that made them think your plan was their idea.*

Shortly after I started working at Rush, my father became ventilator-dependent from chronic obstructive lung disease that had slowly become debilitating. Then, a year before Dad's death, my mother had a stroke and stayed with us in our home until she recovered.

My father, of course, did not survive. One doesn't come back from the level of pulmonary disease he had. After two years of being on a ventilator, he died in 1994.

Fortunately, my mother did very well after about six months of rehabilitation and was able to return to the Oak Lawn home where she still lived.

A bright spot in 1993 was the marriage of John and Clare.

Those years were challenging: a new, very demanding job, frequent visits to my father in his ventilator unit, daily rehabilitation and therapy visits in our home for my mother, and then the need to manage two households, visit Dad, and take Mom to appointments and shopping. John and Bob would have helped, but Bob had left his engineering position at Ford to enter medical school and lived four hours away in a suburb of Detroit. John and Clare lived over an hour away in a far northern suburb of Chicago.

It was during those years that I experienced first-hand being a caregiver for the seriously ill.

Gradually it became apparent that I had a great deal of responsibility. My sons still called me when problems arose, and I wanted to be involved in their lives. I was the one who cared for my parents. My brother would have helped, but he lived in California and had younger children, whereas I lived twenty minutes away and Chris and I were empty nesters. It fell on me, the one who lived nearby. The one who was capable.

In truth, I realized it was my nature to accept responsibility, so I wanted to do as much as I could. Chris was amazingly supportive and took a lot off my shoulders. But there was little time left for "me."

During that time, I discovered that it was physically exhausting and emotionally draining living with the constant worry about whether or not my efforts would produce any results for the people I loved. But there were rewarding moments too, the ones when we appreciated each other, were thankful and happy for our close ties, despite the challenges that were forced on us.

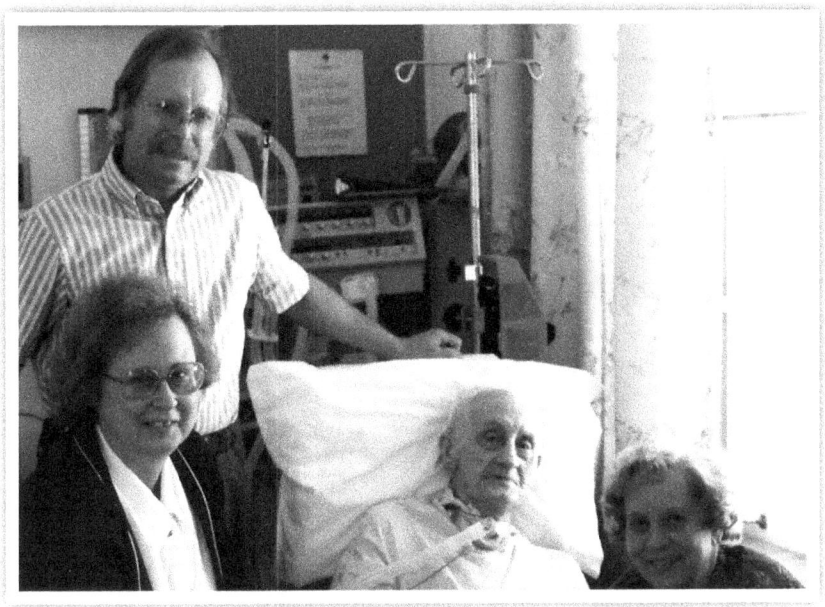

Ventilator Unit: Me, brother Mike, Dad and Mom.

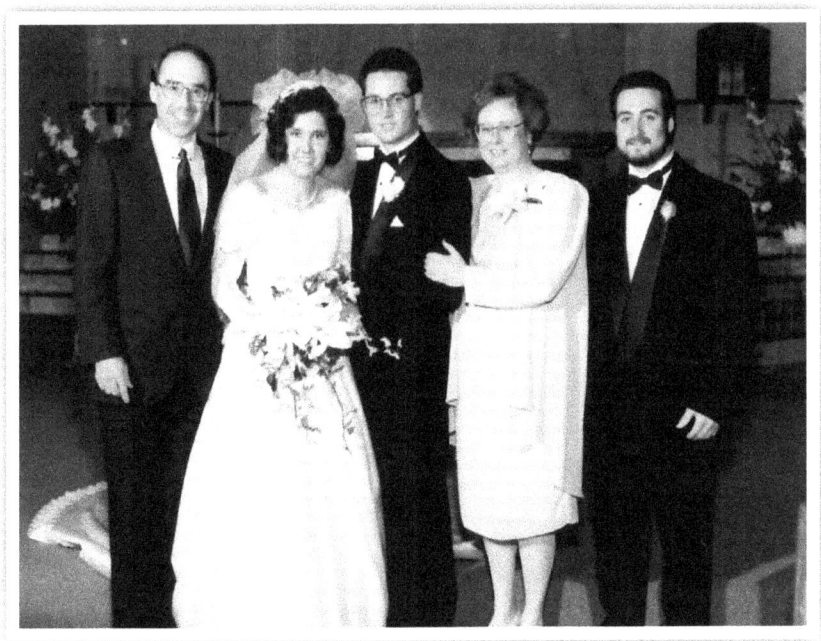

John and Clare's Wedding: Chris, Clare, John, me, and Bob

CHAPTER 28
Preparing for Side Effects
Early January 2018

"The doctor said you had to do something, you had to do it. That's pretty much it. They seemed confident, very polite, so I had confidence in them. I think you had good care, ten on a scale of one to ten." - Chris, husband

I hadn't entirely shaken my doubts that I even had cancer. I felt good. So why was I subjecting myself to treatment that would make me feel bad for months or even longer? Perhaps worse than I had ever felt?

The reason, of course, was that I wanted to be cured. Dying was an option I refused to consider. I was scared of the possibility and didn't want to take any chances. I wanted all existing cancer and any microscopic seeds traveling through my body gone forever and good health restored. I wanted the little dancing shaman to banish the Johnny Appleseed bad guy forever.

I'd worked in the medical field most of my life and learned who to trust. I fully realized I was fortunate to live today instead of twenty years ago when the outcome for my type of cancer was not so good. Today squamous cell cancer of the base of the tongue is one of the more curable types of cancer. For nonsmokers with cancers like mine, survival rates are high.

But the treatment for my kind of cancer is tough. I didn't realize *how* tough it was at the beginning. Not as bad as it used to be, especially with my research trial, but still tough.

As much as I trusted my medical team, I believed that I had to personally cooperate, participate, and manage my disease. This self-reliant attitude was probably instilled in me after being responsible not only for myself but for others for so many years.

Both Cetuximab and radiation therapy are expected to cause various changes during treatment. I was told about common effects before treatment began, and details were included in the literature I had been given.

A very few people experience kidney damage, scarring of the lungs, or shock to the heart. I saw those possibilities as remote, and they didn't concern me much. That's why I chose a major academic center, where they were prepared to deal with such emergencies. I was a bit of a fatalist. I figured if sudden death was in store for me, it was more likely to happen in an accident of some sort. There was nothing I could do about fate, so it would do no good to worry about it.

The literature I read informed me that up to one in five people can experience a serious allergic reaction, faint, get a blood clot, or have bouts of confusion or depression. Those issues didn't worry me much either. I had suffered through emergencies and traumas in the past, and I thought I'd handled them without significant emotional or cognitive issues. I felt confident those problems wouldn't happen to me or I could handle them if they did.

Common effects were the ones that worried me, so I considered those in more detail, so I'd be prepared when they occurred. Here are my early opinions about the effects I expected, how impactful I thought they would be, and what I planned to do about them:

Both Cetuximab and radiation cause skin changes.

It had been many years since I took a degree in biology, but when I read that Cetuximab worked by affecting growth factor receptors in the epidermis of the skin, it made sense that skin effects should be expected. The epidermis is the outer layer of tissue that lines the skin as well as organs and membranes in other parts of the body, such as the mouth. It is composed of epithelial and squamous cells. Squamous cell cancer is what I had. Cancer treatment kills cancer cells, but damages healthy cells too. It seemed likely that my skin would undergo some changes. I certainly wouldn't like them.

I'm of Irish and Polish descent, born blond with fair skin and blue eyes.

My skin has always been sensitive and burns easily. I knew I would be more susceptible to skin changes and had to be more careful than most people. In addition to preparing myself mentally, I took measures to avoid dehydration by drinking more water and using a humidifier next to my bed at night.

At least I didn't have to worry about sun exposure in January. I wouldn't be outdoors in skimpy clothing.

Changes in nails.

Yeah, so what? How awful could bad nails be? If they looked unsightly, they'd grow out. But I cut my nails short, so I didn't have to deal with nail care.

Swelling and redness in areas of radiation.

Okay. A bigger issue, but I'd had burns. Burns hurt pretty bad, but last just so long and there are salves and Tylenol.

Rash, itching, dry skin.

Ditto opinion about burns.

I searched my closets and dresser drawers for soft items with low necks to avoid as much irritation as possible, especially around my neck. I started running my personal laundry and bedding through a second rinse to be sure there was no irritating soap residue. I stopped using liquid cleaners, which are more drying, on my hands, face, and in the shower. Instead, I used a mild bar soap without fragrance or other additives.

I got my hair cut short so hair care products wouldn't irritate my sensitive skin and so I could style it easily.

My nurses gave me skin creams to use proactively to minimize changes so long as I removed them two hours prior to radiation treatments, since creams could cause radiation burns to be worse. I had to avoid wearing anyting below my eyes to mid-chest, since the areas between would be radiated. Even Chapstick was a no-no. Mostly I wore only eye make-up.

I had to forgo the hot showers I loved in favor of warm ones, and I patted my skin dry instead of rubbing it. I must admit that I rewarded myself with a brief, slightly warmer spray on unaffected parts of my body before exiting the shower.

I was told that my appearance would change and that I probably wouldn't want to make public appearances for a while.

Dehydration, weight loss, no appetite.

I could stand to lose some weight. A benefit, not a problem, in my book.

I got a quart-sized drinking container to measure my water intake.

Sores in the mouth and difficulty swallowing.

Okay—that was a concern. Could those problems affect my breathing too? I'd do what I could to avoid that.

Gastrointestinal problems: Constipation, diarrhea, nausea and vomiting.

Those problems were no stranger to me. I thought I could tolerate diarrhea and constipation, and I'd been promised help with the nausea and vomiting. So yeah, one of my main concerns, but I was resigned to tough it out.

Difficulty sleeping, tiredness, headache.

Well, I expected that. I'd nap during the day if necessary. I'd canceled enough activities so I could do that, I thought.

Pain.

I didn't want pain—who does? I also didn't like to take pain medications that made me fuzzy-headed or put me to sleep, and I didn't want to get dependent on them. But hey, I'd take them if I hurt bad enough.

Infection and fever.

Surely medications would be available, and I'd be over it in a few days.

Cough and shortness of breath.

Again, familiar symptoms I could tolerate.

So, I had talked myself into thinking that only a few of these changes were worrisome. I'd pay particular attention to those.

I started, I think, with a good attitude. I'd studied what to expect, and I'd taken steps before problems developed to minimize the side effects.

I didn't think my experience would be as hard for me as it was for others. I knew a lot about medicine, and I had confidence in my doctors and in Rush Medical Center. If I had gone to a community hospital instead of an academic center, I wouldn't have been offered the research study that we were all convinced would save me and be easier than standard care. I was familiar with the hospital and had friends there. I had every intention of cooperating fully with the program. Perhaps I was even a little cocky, but still there was deep worry beneath my conscious thoughts.

I thought I knew what to expect.

Boy, was I wrong! When the problems developed, some of the changes I had initially thought insignificant were surprisingly difficult. I discovered later I couldn't make the changes go away, but I'm sure the methods and precautions I followed made them more livable.

The first side effect I experienced happened in recovery after my tongue biopsy. Whether the extreme secretions immediately after I woke up were due to anesthesia or some other effect of the surgery, the experience was surprisingly distasteful (pun intended!), but fortunately only lasted a couple of hours.

After surgery my only pain was in my throat and just when I swallowed. It was sharp, but much like sore throats I'd had before with respiratory infections. Unlike a respiratory infection, however, I had no other symptoms such as congestion, fever, headache, or cough. So, although uncomfortable, it was tolerable and lessened gradually until I had almost no pain ten days later.

The nausea I had after my first chemotherapy returned only mildly after my second infusion. I was relieved to learn that the premedications seemed to deal with that issue very well. I also never had the extreme muscle weakness and headache I'd experienced after my first infusion again.

The day of, and the morning after, my first radiation treatment, I didn't notice any effect at all from the radiation. I slept reasonably well, and the next morning I ate some breakfast. All my doctors stressed how important good nutrition was, so I forced myself to eat a small serving of oatmeal. I added blueberries, butter, and sugar, two slices of wheat toast, and coffee with creamer, following the advice to consume as many calories as possible.

I stopped in the bathroom after breakfast before leaving the house for my second radiation therapy. My tongue felt a little irritated. I looked at it in the mirror. I was stunned to find that the entire top and sides of my tongue were completely black!

What the hell!

Chris came in from the garage after taking my bag to the car.

"Look at my tongue!" I stuck it out to show him.

He raised his eyebrows. "It's black. Does it hurt?"

I shook my head. "Not at all. It's just black. What do you think that means? Is it from the radiation already?"

"Did they tell you that could happen?"

"No."

"Well, you're going to see them in an hour. Ask them about it."

I rolled my eyes. "Of course I'll ask them about it! You think I'd hide it from them?"

He bit his lower lip and picked up my coat to help me get into it.

In the tomography room, I showed my tongue to Paul. I expected him to laugh and say that this happened all the time. But he drew his eyebrows together. "I've never seen anything like that." He left me seated on the side of the tomography bed and soon the resident radiation oncologist, Dr. Gold, came into the room.

Dr. Gold was a quiet, slender man of about thirty who was already balding. I liked him as soon as I met him. After showing him my tongue, he looked as baffled as Paul.

"This can't be from radiation, but I'm at a loss to explain it. Let me check."

I proceeded with my treatment, and when it was over Dr. Gold came back into the room. He was avoiding my eyes, and I thought he might have been biting his cheeks.

"You said you had oatmeal with blueberries for breakfast, right?" he asked.

I nodded.

"Were the blueberries frozen?"

It was my turn to look baffled. "They were. How did you know?"

As it turned out, little sacs in blueberries contain molecules that make them blue. Freezing breaks the sacs and releases the dye, which can stain the tongue. This does not happen when they're fresh, and the "milk" stays white.

I became known for a time in the radiation therapy department as "The Lady with the Dreaded Blueberry Disease."

I wondered if that condition was covered by Medicare…

CHAPTER 29

Life Before Cancer: Successful Years, 1998-2007

*I*n 1998, during a lull between family medical issues, Chris and I bought a two-story Georgian home, our "dream" house, and moved about twelve miles farther southwest to Lemont. The house was on a half-acre lot. It had a library for all my books, plus four bedrooms and a full basement. We had plenty of room, and we immediately told my mother she was welcome whenever she wanted to move in with us.

Lemont turned out to be a good choice for many reasons. It's set apart from other suburbs, surrounded by forests, farms, and the Des Plaines River Valley. The pace is slower, more relaxing, an escape from a hectic world, with plenty of places to get lost in nature. We were privileged to live in this environment, yet it was only a short distance from anything we wanted in the city. We soon realized it was even more than we had expected at first.

My mother wanted to stay in her home, so Chris and I continued to travel back and forth between our home in Lemont and hers in Oak Lawn so she could live independently as she wished. It was the best decision for her, but it was hard on Chris and me, traveling a half hour each way to take care of her house and take her shopping and to appointments on a frequent basis while we held down demanding jobs.

Happily, two grandsons joined our family, sons of John and Clare. Collin was born in 1999 and Aidan in 2004. It was hard to be a grandma when I lived over an hour away and had a demanding job, but I tried, remembering how much my grandmothers had meant to me when I was a child.

Through all this time, I found my career as administrator of the general surgery practice at Rush very fulfilling. I loved my work. When asked what my job was about, I would answer that I made it possible for important people to do important things. I was proud of what I did, but especially after I added a long commute each day, I had little time for personal pursuits.

Through all the busy and sometimes stressful years, my salvation, my port in the storm, the single thing that kept me going, kept me smiling on those days when a new medical crisis struck my mom or when I regretted the little time I had left for my children and grandchildren, was reading. I had never lost the love for reading that had been with me since I was a child. Although there was less time, a book still was at hand every moment of every day, ready for the rare moments I could open the pages and escape through the words and the worlds of someone else.

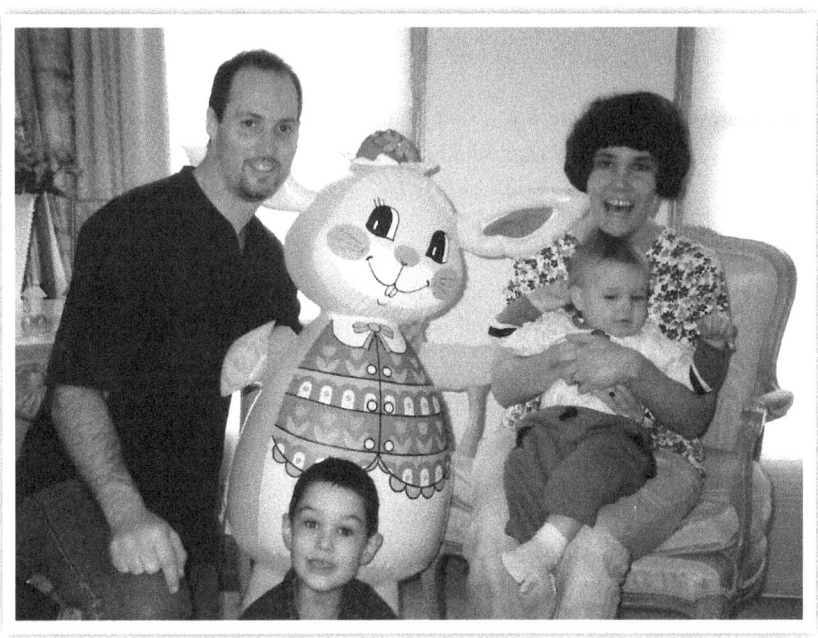

John, Collin, Clare, and Aidan with Big Bunny, Easter 2005.
This is the same bunny John and Bob had as preschoolers.

CHAPTER 30
My First Side Effects
January 2018

"You were talking fine, got in and out of the car by yourself, so I knew you weren't seriously ill. You just had to get rid of the cancer." - Chris, husband

"I was amazed at the steps you had to take to be able to eat. Also, about your schedule, taking medicines and doing all the things you had to do every day was a challenge." - Clare, daughter-in-law

It wasn't long before my daily trips to the hospital settled into a routine. Radiation oncology had scheduled all my daily appointments for one in the afternoon, which allowed Chris and me to leave home about 11:45 a.m. and avoid the morning rush hour. I was usually taken as soon as I arrived. If I needed to see a doctor, dietitian, or therapist, I would see them after my radiation treatment in an exam room in the same department. Usually, we left for home before two in the afternoon, thankfully before the afternoon rush hour started. With travel time, the appointments took three to four hours out of the middle of each day, but that was about as convenient as possible, so we were grateful for the thoughtful scheduling we were offered.

Of course, Thursdays, when I also had to see Dr. Fidler and have an infusion, appointments took the entire day.

When my name was called in radiation oncology, I'd go through automatic double doors into the department, skip the dressing room and continue past other treatment rooms and the rooms where the physicists and dosimetrists made their calculations, and into my treatment room.

I wore a sleeveless scoop-neck cotton tank top that could stay on during the treatment and no bra. After I slipped off my outerwear, Vani would help me onto the table. Paul would come in and we'd chat for a few minutes. Then I'd lie down on my back on the table and Vani and Paul would clamp my mask on both sides, fixing me tightly to the table. Vani would spread a warm blanket over me. Then both therapists would leave and go into the control room.

After a new CT was taken, I'd wait a few minutes for the therapists to match the areas to be treated to the scan. Then in a few minutes, I'd hear the treatment machine start humming, warming up. Paul would tell me over the loudspeaker that we were ready to begin. The humming and whirring would increase in intensity, the table would draw me upward into the bore, and soon the rattling that reminded me of a Native American medicine man would begin. When I asked about the sound, Paul told me it was caused by the opening and closing of gears in the bore that directed the beams to each precise programmed location in my treatment zone.

I never used the breathing and relaxation techniques I had practiced. As I lay bolted to the table with radiation beaming through me, confined and motionless, I preferred to say prayers to pass the time. I would repeat the Our Father, Hail Mary, and Glory Be, as if I were counting sheep. I said each series of prayers, matching the cadence to the rhythm of my heartbeat, slow and regular. The routine regulated my heart and breathing rates. I counted the repetitions on my fingers, and between each I prayed that my cancer would be cured. Making prayers a routine helped me determine how much longer I had before the treatment was finished, since I learned that after seven repetitions, the rattling would stop.

I was usually in the treatment room less than half an hour. In the car on the way home I would eat some lunch and do a round of speech therapy exercises.

Many patients have the same diagnosis of squamous cell tongue cancer, but that doesn't mean that every patient will have the same treatment, the same reactions, or the same results. Even if the treatment were the same, everyone reacts differently to chemotherapy and radiation therapy. Some side effects are a major problem for one patient, but another patient doesn't have that problem at all.

I can only tell my own story and speak about the problems I experienced and what I learned about the problems I feared but *didn't* have. Based on what my doctors told me, my treatment was easier than most. That could be due to my cooperation with their suggestions and the research study option that minimized side effects.

Nonetheless, before long I began noticing side effects and recording them in my journal. I thought I was getting off lightly at first, but it didn't last.

Early in January, happy that I had escaped the dreaded nausea, so far at least, I soon discovered I had to deal with constipation. It could have been caused by chemotherapy, but more likely it was because I was eating less food and different food.

I had been on multiple medications before I got cancer, and now a bedroom table held an overflowing shoe box full of new pills, creams, salves, and mouth rinses to be taken either prophylactically, regularly, or as needed when symptoms developed. I hated the idea of being dependent on prescriptions. I wanted to limit what I was taking, which included anything for constipation. So I decided to try prunes. I added both prune juice and prunes to my schedule, hoping that would take care of the problem.

Then a few days later I had to stop eating prunes because I developed diarrhea. That caused such severe anal irritation that I had to skip a few of my daily walks. That was no good. Regular exercise was important to keep me fit, maintain strength, and prevent muscle loss during therapy. Humiliatingly, I had to start using diaper cream. I pulled out my schedule again and added diaper cream applications.

When treatment began, my nurses told me that both Cetuximab and radiation would cause changes to my skin and mucous membranes. I reminded myself that both mucous membranes and skin are composed of the same type of cells and are susceptible to the same changes. The lining of the entire gastrointestinal tract (esophagus, stomach, etc.), including the mouth, are covered with mucous membranes. Most patients who have chemotherapy and/or radiation therapy for head and neck cancer suffer some GI effects.

Robbie, my radiation therapy nurse, had told me during my first appointment that mucositis was likely.

"Mucositis covers the mouth with a sticky layer of secretions. It causes saliva to be thick and difficult to swallow or spit out. Your mouth may look slimy, either white or red, and you can develop sores that might make not only your mouth but your throat raw, burning, and painful and make swallowing food harder. It will likely also affect your esophagus."

He paused and searched my eyes, probably to be sure I appreciated the importance of his instructions.

"Mucositis can last not only throughout your therapy, but up to three months after therapy's finished. But it's not permanent. It will eventually go away completely."

He gave me a sample of MuGard then and told me to start using it right away to keep mucositis to a minimum.

I used it like he told me to, but I was unconvinced. I hated MuGard from the first time I tried it. Yuk! It was like rinsing with syrup and left a sickly-sweet taste in my mouth that lasted for hours. Four times a day, and I had to wait thirty minutes before I could put anything else in my mouth to kill the unpleasantness. I didn't at that time have any symptoms of mucositis, so the additional rinse didn't seem important to me at the time.

Although using MuGard to *prevent* mucositis was logical, its importance got lost in the vast array of everything that was happening. Even though I was clearly told to expect this problem, there was so much going on that seemed more important at the time. I selected some problems to focus on and put others out of my mind to deal with later. Mucositis was one of the problems I underrated.

Near the beginning of treatment, I thought I had broken a couple of teeth or jarred a filling out of place because whenever my tongue passed over certain teeth, they felt unusually sharp. After a few days I realized my tongue was so sensitive that all tooth surfaces felt sharp. I gradually got used to this.

By the second week of treatment, I began to tolerate fewer and fewer foods. Nothing tasted good. Most foods either hurt my mouth or made me nauseous. I felt full all the time, and after a few bites of food I felt stuffed and bloated. Eating became a serious concern. Anything that made eating more difficult was sure to have an impact on my ability to stick it out to the end.

Later that same week I started having a dry mouth and taste changes. I couldn't eat anything dry, like bread or crackers, and if I didn't keep moving my mouth it felt like my mouth was sticking together. After chewing for a while, I had to add water to what was in my mouth to be able to swallow. Otherwise the food would cling to the back of my throat, and I couldn't swallow it.

Eating became an adventure. Everything I put in my mouth was a surprise—not always unpleasant, just different. When I expected something sweet, it was salty. Salty things might taste sweet or bland. Peanut butter might taste like applesauce, applesauce might taste like eggs. I'd be prepared for a particular taste—I didn't lose my ability to smell—but never knew what I was going to get. It was like a game.

Impossible to avoid bad weather in January in Chicago. On Sunday, January 14, it started to snow at night and didn't stop until noon on Tuesday. Fortunately, the thirty-mile one-way trips to the hospital took place outside of rush hour and traffic was only a little worse than normal.

About two weeks after therapy began, I started to have an "underwater" feeling, as if my ears were plugged, followed in the next two days by tenderness and then a clear discharge from my left ear.

My ENT was able to see me the same day I called. I wanted to tell him we had to stop meeting like this, but I held my tongue. "What's going on with my ear?" I asked instead.

He confirmed that my left ear was inflamed. He explained that my throat and other internal structures were experiencing burns internally similar to what I would see on my neck externally, and the swelling and inflammation were affecting my ears. He was concerned with what he saw. I was given an antibiotic and eardrops. The problem cleared up after about a week and never returned.

Wednesday, January 24, after two weeks of radiation and three infusions, I developed the first symptoms of mucositis. When I woke up that morning the entire lining of my mouth was mildly sore: cheeks, tongue, gums, throat—all of it. I had a raw sore on my tongue that made it hard to chew without pain.

What had been predicted was beginning.

By then I had lost what little of my appetite remained. I ate not for pleasure, not due to hunger, but because I had to. Gradually more foods got less appealing, and I began limiting my choices. I had been eating hard-boiled eggs and biscuits for lunch every day. I thought I'd try egg salad one day. The mayonnaise tasted rancid. The same unpleasantness persisted with other foods I tried. I picked foods least likely to taste bad, and ended up eventually with only oatmeal, scrambled eggs, creamed soups, Ensure, cottage cheese, and pudding.

One night I woke up with a feeling of pressure and thickness at the back of my throat and across my windpipe that made breathing seem more difficult. I panicked.

Oh please, I thought, *let me breathe!* In the middle of the night sensations often seem out of proportion, life-threatening. More difficult is a relative term. My mind worked on me. Was I breathing normally? Consciously, no. Was it *difficult* to breathe? No. Not really. But worrying about whether or not I could breathe scared me, nonetheless. I had visions of my throat swelling and my airway being cut off. The sensation was vague, but the potential frightening. It seemed that I was getting less air, but fear will do that to you. When I continued to take air in and out, I gradually calmed myself enough to fall back to sleep.

When I went for radiation therapy the next day, Dr. Gold examined and then reassured me. Yes, there was some swelling, but nothing unexpected. It would be highly unusual for radiation changes to impact my airway. With this reassurance, I got used to the feeling and after a while I no longer noticed it.

By Friday, two days later and three weeks after my first infusion, I developed more sores inside my cheeks.

"I keep biting my tongue, the sides of my cheeks, and these sores," I complained to Dr. Gold.

"That's because radiation has altered the usual sensations in your mouth. Since you were a baby, you trained your mouth to react to its customary sensations, but now the sensations are different and the training is lost. How badly are you chewing them?" he asked.

"Once I bite an area hard, I'm careful. The sore will heal in a day or two if I don't bite it again. But then I'll bite a new spot."

"There's nothing that will stop that from happening except being careful, like you're doing. It doesn't sound like we have to treat you for infection. How about the pain? You can take some of your pain pills if you need to."

I still wanted to save the pain medicines for when I might really need them. I didn't want to develop dependency on them. I was also afraid if I took tramadol before I really needed to, it wouldn't be as effective if I had serious pain down the road.

"The pain is only when I aggravate the area too much. I'll just be careful. I think I can handle this."

"Okay but remember that your sleep and your nutrition are very important. Don't sacrifice those to pain. If you need medication, take it."

Then skin changes began. My face and neck became dry and itchy. I increased the amount of the sample lotion I'd been given and the number of times a day I used it, but this had no effect.

Dr. Fidler told me I had developed what is called a "Cetuximab rash" on the back of my neck. Apparently, ninety percent of patients on Cetuximab develop an acne-like rash on the face, neck, back, chest, or arms. I had been given steroid and antibiotic creams to treat the rash when it occurred, so I started using the steroid cream.

Being January, it was impossible to avoid wearing fabric near the rash on the back of my neck, but I did my best. I wore V-neck and low-neck tops backward, away from areas of rash.

I wasn't prepared for how itchy the rash would be, though. Of course, scratching would irritate the rash even more, so getting the itching under control required another medication. I couldn't use hot or cold packs on the rash either. So I toughed it out. It felt especially itchy in bed at night, as I lay there with little to think about except my body and my worries.

Next, I noticed a painful hangnail, and the skin on my fingertips started to split, like small paper cuts that would not heal. But these cuts were considerably more painful than paper cuts. It became hard to do anything that required the use of the tips of my fingers, such as typing or preparing meals.

The splits on my fingers, and later on my feet, could be excruciating. If I avoided touching them I didn't have pain—until I forgot and touched them accidentally—which seemed to happen way too often.

That weekend, I had a significant drop in my energy level. On Saturday, I noticed that, instead of tasting weird, my food seemed to have less taste.

By Sunday, the end of my first month of therapy, the ability to distinguish between flavors was suddenly completely gone. Everything I put in my mouth tasted the same, metallic and salty, even water. Eventually, I could eat only oatmeal and Ensure.

The secretions in my mouth were becoming thick and nauseating. These secretions, I learned, were not saliva but caused by the slimy covering in my mouth from mucositis. I had to use Zofran (my nausea medication) regularly. The back of my throat, tongue, and soft palate felt swollen and tender. Soon I had to start taking pain medications (mostly Tylenol) regularly as well.

It was even harder to eat because I had no appetite at all, and tasteless food felt strange in my mouth. I could chew and swallow automatically, but all the pleasure and satisfaction of eating were gone. I felt miserable, with the itchy neck I couldn't scratch, the painful fingers, and I was so tired I didn't feel like doing anything but sitting in a chair. It was even hard to summon enough energy to read.

In just a few days I had gone from celebrating an easy ride to acknowledging that I wasn't going to escape unscathed. At this point, I wondered how bad my side effects would get. I could get through my day on my own when I had to. I didn't have significant pain, only bothersome. But it was becoming more difficult to do anything except keep my appointments and attempt to do everything on my checklist.

Yet I was determined to do whatever I could to minimize the inevitable.

What was discouraging was that up to then I thought I was *already* doing everything I'd been advised to do, but I was suffering all these symptoms anyway. When you're doing everything you can, it's normal to expect that you will stop bad things from happening and get better. I had to adjust my thinking along the lines of "not as bad as it would be if you didn't do everything you could."

What is "everything" anyway? Isn't there always something else that can be done if you look hard enough? Maybe the times I skipped or was prevented from completing my daily list by some interference caused this symptom. Or maybe I wasn't using enough of the medicines, or doing my therapy exercises long enough or often enough. Was I really doing *everything* I could?

I thought so. I really did. As much, so they say, as was humanly possible. As humanly possible for *me*!

I remembered again my mother's words when she was struggling with end-of-life challenges: "Staying alive is a lot of work!"

Perhaps I needed an attitude adjustment.

By Tuesday, thick secretions coated every surface in my mouth. I had a continuous urge to swallow and remove the "gunk," as I called it, but it was too thick to swallow completely. The more I swallowed, the more my mouth produced. The unpleasant, nauseating gunk gathered at the back of my throat.

By Wednesday, the last day of the first month of therapy, my neck was not only itchy but tender to touch. It was hard to eat. I needed to nap to get through the day. That day I couldn't take a daily walk, and from that time on I discontinued walking.

Prior to being diagnosed with cancer, I had done a vast amount of research and had begun writing my third historical mystery novel, *The Mystery at Mount Forest Island*. I didn't think I could write a good story when I was so consumed by my health. I had set aside the book for a better time. I did, however, think that writing was something I could still do. If taken in small bits, I could sit at a computer for brief periods a few days a week and continue posting to the local history blog I had created to promote my books. I didn't feel up to researching local history, but I would write about my experiences with cancer.

Writing my blog would serve several purposes. It would distract me from thinking about how miserable I felt and give me a manageable goal. It would serve as a way to look closely but objectively at my experience and preserve the record for myself, my doctors, and my family. It would keep me in touch with my fans while I was unable to interact with them in other ways. And I felt I was a good person to inform other cancer patients due to my combination of experiences with medicine, writing, and the disease.

On January 30, 2018, I published my first blog post about my experience with cancer: "My Personal Journey Through Head and Neck Cancer." This post told my followers how I found out I had cancer, how I wrestled with doubts about the diagnosis, and how I decided to enroll in a clinical trial.

And so ended January, my first month of chemotherapy, and my first three weeks of radiation therapy. I started the month relatively comfortable, questioning my diagnosis although trusting my doctors to guide me. By the end of the month, I found myself surprised by the full magnitude of cancer treatment. The days ahead were going to be worse than I had optimistically thought. No matter how much I did to minimize those effects, it was going to be hard to finish.

On the other hand, I was grateful that my background in medicine and my general good health at the beginning allowed me to have a good attitude. I was a cooperative patient, and I was likely to suffer less than many patients with the same cancer.

Cooperation, following the rules, doing things the right way, were all part of my nature. I was the sort of person who read every word of the directions and would come to a full stop at a stop sign even if it was two in the morning in the middle of nowhere without another car or person in sight. I'd use my turn signal in the same circumstances.

Yet, at this point, I found myself questioning whether the cure was worse than the disease.

CHAPTER 31
First Month of Treatment Ends

"I was concerned about all the things you had to go through, but I approved of what the doctors were doing and the decisions you made."
– Chris, husband

"When we talked about your plan and your medications, I was very thankful that you had the mental faculties to manage things." – Clare, daughter-in-law

I had finished the first full month of my cancer treatment.

I had another month to go.

Another month when I could expect my side effects to build in intensity.

I had established routines. There was comfort in the familiar surroundings as well as in the feeling of accomplishment for having gotten this far without a major setback. I was still able to walk into the hospital on my own. We didn't need to make any changes to my treatment plan.

Although there had been unpleasant surprises, I was encouraged by the thought that, so far at least, nothing struck me as unbearable. The intensity of side effects hadn't been much greater than problems caused by illnesses or injuries I'd had in the past.

The major difference that made my life so hard was the cumulative effect of so many problems happening at once and increasing fatigue and weakness. Coupled with that, these problems went on and on, week after week, with no way of knowing when, or if, I would get better. I tried to convince myself that I'd gotten this far, so I could stand another month. I didn't think past that.

Halfway there, the end in sight.

By the beginning of February, aside from my trips to the hospital, I was spending almost all my time at home. My family and friends sent cards and gifts, offered prayers, and called me frequently. I kept most conversations short. I was tired and, rather than rehashing my medical experiences, even with family and close friends, I was more interested in distractions: reading, watching television, or sleeping. Carolyn, a close friend since sixth grade who now lived in northwestern Iowa, wanted to come to visit, but I discouraged her. Much as I would have loved to see her and was thrilled that she offered, I knew I didn't have the energy to host a house guest.

Others wanted to visit and offered to cook meals for us. I appreciated their offers, but I needed to rest more, and there were so few foods I could eat. I continued to cook for Chris and accepted a few meal offers for him, but for me? I could hardly say, "Much as I'd love your lasagna, could you bring me a bowl of oatmeal?"

By February, even phone calls were hard to manage. I needed plenty of sleep, so I didn't get up until after eight in the morning. By the time I took pills, prepared and struggled to eat breakfast, and did all my morning routines, it was time to leave for radiation therapy. When I returned from the hospital by late midafternoon most days, there were routines to check off. I was often too tired to do much except nap. My relationships with family and friends, although their good wishes were appreciated, were strained.

I was tired of making up reassuring answers to "How are you doing today?" when I felt like shit. One well-meaning friend insisted that marijuana was the answer to my problems and got argumentative when I said that could be true, but I didn't care to try it.

All I wanted to hear was sentiments like, "I'm thinking about you and wishing you didn't have to go through this." Or "I know it must be hard. If you want to talk, I'm here any time."

An exception to my wishes for short calls was my immediate family. I talked regularly with Bob and Dolly, who were always available for medical advice as well as moral support. John also called me regularly to find out how I was doing and to encourage me.

Clare recognized my exhaustion and sent me a lovely card she had made for me that included an iPhone charger cord, an adapter for me to use during hospital visits, and a note. In part, the note said:

> *"John called you today and I am thankful he is calling you often. I worry that you may be tired of talking, so I hope this note will let you know that I would love to talk to you too and that it is nice to get a card in the mail. I hope to encourage you to keep your spirits up. Think about those little things that give you happiness and give yourself permission to do them. Find your happy things and pull them out to cheer you up.*
>
> *"I am thankful that at this time you have a loving, giving husband, a small and loving family, good friends, and family only an hour away. You are a fighter, you have family with great medical knowledge, and connections from your own career. I am thankful for modern medicine and how it can help you get well.*
>
> *"I like to make a card because I spend the time away from distractions and pray for whomever I am making the card for. Maybe you just want to know I think of you while I create a card. I hope you know it is filled with love!"*

Another exception to short phone calls was my best friend, Dorothy. Since high school days we had always shared every experience, good or bad. Most of the time we talked on the phone because after we were both married we never lived close to each other.

We managed to fit in a call now and then, either before I left for the hospital or in the late afternoon. These calls were important to me. I never had to pretend to be brave or that things were better than they really were when talking to Dorothy. Nor did I have to listen to well-meaning but repetitive words of encouragement or suggestions I knew wouldn't work for me. With Dorothy, I could unburden myself. I could cry if I wanted to, but instead, no matter how tough things got, we were always able to share a much-needed laugh. Positive thinking is a real challenge for a chronic worrier like me, so these moments of humor were uplifting.

I had complained to Dorothy about how the skin on my hands was so dry, thin, and wrinkled that anything I touched that had an edge was painful.

A few days later, I told her, "Your idea about the Vaseline and gloves worked like a charm."

"Huh! You actually tried that?" she said. "I was joking."

"Yeah, I remembered I had some old vintage gloves somewhere in the basement. I was going to take them to an antique shop, but I couldn't get the stains out."

"Why didn't you throw them away?" Dorothy asked.

"Who knows? Because they were old, I guess. I thought they had to be worth something to someone." Dorothy had no problem pitching things. I, on the other hand, was more than happy to *give* things away, but struggled to throw out anything that *should* have a use—even if it didn't.

"I guess you were right to save something this time."

"I'm right about one time out of twenty."

"That many times? Be honest."

We laughed.

"Anyway, I did what you said, rubbed Vaseline on my hands and put the gloves on before bedtime and slept in them. Thin cotton gloves, like you said, not knit or leather. It worked so well I even wear them during the day sometimes."

"Are you wearing a house dress now, too? A babushka tied around your head?"

"No, but I can't un-see that now," I said.

After we stopped laughing, I added, "With the gloves on, I can open containers and push down on a knife hard enough to cut things. I can even type in them, and my keyboard doesn't get slimy with hand cream."

"Now I can't un-see that," she said.

Sometimes when we talked, we got to laughing so hard it was minutes before we could resume a conversation. I really needed that. Dorothy was the perfect person to understand how much a little personal triumph meant and to celebrate in the telling.

February 4 was the Super Bowl. Although I liked football, I had little interest in the game that year since the Chicago Bears finished last in their division. Chris, however, enjoyed football no matter which teams were playing. I pretended interest and dozed while he had an opportunity to do something he liked for a change, watching the Philadelphia Eagles defeat the New England Patriots.

The following day, February 5, 2018, the stock market crashed. The Dow plunged 1413 points, the greatest point drop ever, and immediately the plunge spread worldwide. There was little that could be done to protect our lifetime savings and IRA investments. We would just have to pray for a recovery of the market, as we were already praying for *my* recovery. Another blow that came at a bad time, but I was too involved in the greater issue of my health. We would have to worry about our financial health after my physical health returned.

Each morning I would finish my medical routines, then try to squeeze in a personal task, such as paying bills or writing my blog. Then Chris and I set out for the daily trip to the hospital, and when I returned in mid to late afternoon, I was too tired to do much more than complete another round of medical routines and make something for dinner. After dinner, I'd drag myself to the family room and try to stay awake in front of the television.

February 9 the 23rd Winter Olympics opened in South Korea. I had only moderate interest, but the Olympics turned out to be the perfect distraction. The opening and closing ceremonies, like all Olympics, were lengthy but had spectacular visual effects, musical performances, and an impressive number of participants. The Olympics were on just about any time I cared to tune in, and of course I hoped for the Americans to do well, especially in figure skating.

I admired the athletes but envied them a bit. I had little athletic talent. I had ice skated a little when I was still in grade school, but my ankles were never strong enough to keep me from doing more than wobbling around a frozen pond, and the cold got to me. I did, however, remember the exhilaration of gliding over ice, and the combination of that memory, hearing the music, and watching the Olympic performances gave me almost as much joy as choral singing.

The United States didn't take many skating metals that year. My memory of details is poor, due to personal worry and fatigue. I cared enough to be interested in an event, but not enough that I felt like I missed something when I fell asleep during a competition I had wanted to see, and I did exactly that most nights. I was vaguely aware of other events such as bobsled, downhill skiing, speed skating, and ski jumping. I do remember Shaun White taking gold again for the third time in the halfpipe. Although, truth be told, I didn't see a whole lot of sense in that particular event.

Since all the channels we usually watched were showing reruns during the Olympics, all in all, the Olympics running during my treatment was a gift that helped keep my mind occupied and helped me relax at a tough time.

CHAPTER 32

Life Before Cancer: New Personal Activities, 2003-2008

*M*edical administration was personally rewarding, but I laughingly told everyone that what I actually did was write all day long. I wrote letters, correspondence, memos, procedures, reports, web content, minutes. And my philosophy was, if I expected anyone to read what I wrote and to follow the advice or instructions I was giving, my written words had to be accurate, clear, easy to understand, and if possible entertaining. So I learned to write that way, and I guess I had a knack for writing as well as administration, because I was frequently told, "You should write a book."

That comment was tempting, but impossible. Medical administration was a 24/7 job. True, I made time to read and listen to books on tape while driving to and from work between Lemont and the Medical District in Chicago each day. But writing a novel myself was another matter. So I put it off, still not seriously thinking I could be a writer.

Raised by parents with modest expectations, I lacked confidence. I had a successful career in medical administration, but writers were something else. Writers were celebrities! A different matter entirely.

As retirement approached, I asked myself again when it would be "my time." Was I going to work after the normal retirement age of sixty-five? Or was

I going to retire and give in at last to the lure of doing what I wanted? I knew I couldn't do both.

I loved my career. I felt important. I went to work every day believing I helped important people save lives. I felt proud of what I'd done. But what about more personal things? What exactly were those unfulfilled dreams? What might my life be like once my career was over?

As a lifelong workaholic, I was worried that I wouldn't have enough to do after I retired. I had seen too many people laze around and grow feeble due to lack of interests and activities and die too young. I didn't want that to happen. But did I want to work long into retirement? Or did I want to pursue interests I'd put off all my life?

I started to actively think about putting my feet in the water right away, to try out things that would fill my life after I retired.

I was already enjoying my newfound love for our town of Lemont, walking the I&M Canal and the forest preserve trails. Retirement would give me more time to do that.

In 2003, Chris had found an ad in the local paper asking for candidates to fill vacancies on the Lemont Public Library District board. He urged me to interview for one of the appointments. I did so and was honored to be selected as one of the new library board members.

I had enjoyed singing in choral groups since high school, and whenever I could, I sang with church choirs, but I hadn't been with a choir that sang the classical music I loved for years.

Chris ran across an ad in a local paper again, this time asking for new members of a classical chorus that sang in a nearby suburb. Knowing how important singing was to me, he persuaded me to try out. I did, and to my delight was accepted as a member of the Downers Grove Choral Society in late 2005.

I began those activities first. And then I retired from medical administration.

CHAPTER 33
Second Month of Treatment
February 2018

"Half the people who came into the waiting room had wheelchairs or walkers, but you walked in and out, so I figured you can't be that bad. You were tired, but you seemed to be doing better than most people. You weren't in a wheelchair. I didn't have to carry you. You did it all on your own."
- Chris, husband

As February progressed, so did the changes in my mouth and skin. My rash spread to my chest, fortunately to a lesser extent than on my neck. The rash stayed with me throughout treatment. At the same time as the rash, I lost hair at my neckline. I didn't lose any other hair, but my hair did become brittle, coarse, and dry. My eyelashes, which had always been long and thick, became thin and short, but I didn't lose them completely.

Now the skin on my face also became very dry. My cheeks and chin were bright red and raw. Then my elbows, then the tops of my feet and my ankles. I developed painful cracks in the creases behind my heels and could no longer wear shoes with backs.

The painful splits on my fingers also continued. I found that covering my fingertips with a bandage stopped the pain, but each split took a couple of weeks to heal, and by then I had more of them. Dr. Fidler suggested the use of liquid bandage, and that was easier to work with, although each split still lasted a week or more and I usually had two to five going at a time.

The skin lotions I had been using began to burn, so I changed to a thick cream that was free of alcohol, dyes, fragrances, etc. It was a gift sent to me by Clare, my daughter-in-law. The brand she sent was Vanicream. It was better than other products and didn't burn.

My fingertips became furrowed and waxy. This wasn't uncomfortable, just strange, like working with thin gloves I couldn't take off or fingers covered with dry glue. It became hard to grip well or turn pages, and my iPhone no longer recognized my thumbprint. I had to ask Chris to help me open and close zippers, take the tops off pill bottles or food containers, and turn lamp switches. This continued through the entire course of my therapy and afterward.

During the last few weeks of infusions, I had learned techniques to alleviate these symptoms as much as possible, but then the remaining skin on my body started to claim equal attention. The skin on my arms, upper legs, buttocks, and back started to roughen and develop a snakeskin or fish scale texture.

"Look at this," I told Chris, lifting my nightshirt and revealing my upper thigh. "Who ever thought chemotherapy would do something like this?"

"Does it hurt?" he asked, eyeing my leg skeptically.

"No. But when I run my hand over my skin, it doesn't feel like me. It's like I'm turning into some creature. Snakewoman maybe."

"What superpowers would go along with that?" he asked with a grin.

"Maybe I could sneak up on a bad guy, coil around him, and swallow him whole."

"I'll be afraid to sleep in the same bed with you now," he said, slipping under the covers.

I got into bed, curled up against him, and said, "Ssssss..."

About the same time, I started to develop a waxy texture on the bottoms of my feet, similar to what had happened to my fingertips. I got some minor cracking there too and intensified my foot care by adding foot cream daily. The waxy texture made it slippery to walk in bare feet. I had to be very careful not to fall, especially when taking a shower. A warm shower since I still couldn't tolerate hot water on my skin.

These effects were surprising and annoying, but not seriously troublesome or greatly painful. I threw my hands up at yet another insult and tried to convince myself I'd return to normal eventually.

Then my tongue became even more sensitive on both sides and on its surface. In the mirror, it was red and had an ugly deep furrow down the center. I read that some patients reported feeling like their tongue was going to burst, but mine never got that bad.

At the same time, I started to have considerable discomfort in the lining of my nose. Dry crusts covered both nostrils, and when I blew my nose the patches would break off and bleed. I also had occasional nosebleeds. I remembered that all membranes, or linings, could be affected by my treatment, as well as by expected dehydration. I turned up the humidifier and the nosebleeds stopped, but the crusting continued.

On February 9 there was another snowstorm. It started on Thursday night, and all radiation therapy appointments were canceled Friday. The storm turned out to be a gift for me since it gave me a long weekend at a difficult time. I received a double treatment one day the following week, so there was no inconvenience or any effect on my treatment plan.

Up to that point, most of my side effects were due to chemotherapy. About two weeks before my last radiation therapy session, in mid-February, I started to get radiation burns in the treatment area. The burns spread and increased in severity until the back of my neck was extremely raw and irritated. It looked awful—red and blistered. At first it felt like a bad sunburn, which most of us have had at one time or another. I thought I could get through it.

Like any burn, the area was tender and itchy. I was advised to use a silver ointment twice a day that had an antibiotic in it. I also soaked the area with a prescribed solution three times a day, which had a soothing effect. Between those treatments I smoothed on Vanicream every two hours during waking hours. As a result, I was more comfortable during the day, but itching kept me up at night. After a while, I found that Aquaphor had a more healing effect through the night.

Some burns are only painful, but a burn that is both painful and itchy takes discomfort to another level. It's hard not to rub or scratch the itch, which increases the intensity of the pain. The pain and the itch war with each other for top man on the totem pole, and relief is hard to bring about.

I've always been conservative about taking pills for pain, but it was important to get enough rest. My doctors had encouraged me not to deny myself pain meds, so I started to use them with caution. At first, I took only Tylenol before going to bed. Then throat and mouth pain started to get increasingly severe throughout the day, so I took Tylenol at seven in the morning and two in the afternoon, and Norco at bedtime. Pain meds made me more comfortable but didn't help swallowing pain. Oddly, swallowing itself did help temporarily. My throat pain decreased soon after I started eating but returned as soon as I stopped. My aversion to food, however, stuck with me.

At that time, four to five weeks into treatment, my mouth side effects got really bad. I consulted Robbie, my radiation oncology nurse.

"There's got to be something more I can do," I complained.

Robbie gave me a detailed and clearer understanding of what each product I used was meant to do.

"Your symptoms are what we call multifactorial—a combination of problems with different causes, so to speak. Therefore, you need to use each product for the symptom it's meant to fix, as no single product will address all your problems. So, let's take the symptoms one at a time.

"Saltwater rinses are effective to thin the thick secretions you have in your mouth and make it easier to spit them out. So gargle with salt, the more frequently the better. At least four to six times a day, for at least a half minute, and then spit it out."

"Um...how do I make a salt rinse?" I asked.

"One teaspoon of salt and one tablespoon of baking soda in a quart of warm water. After you use it, spit out as much of the secretions as you can without straining. Then don't put anything in your mouth for at least a half hour. You could also try Robitussin, which you can buy over the counter. Some patients think that helps."

I jotted down the recipe and instructions, thinking about adding another six lines to my daily schedule, which already ran onto a second page.

"Now about the MuGard. You've told me you don't like it, but it will help prevent mouth sores and could calm down the *production* of the secretions. It's the only product we have that does that, so try it again. Do you still have any of the bottle I gave you?"

"Yes, Dr. Gold told me that too. But that bottle won't last long at the rate

I'm supposed to use it."

"I can give you more sample bottles, but I'm sorry, you're likely to run out of it. Unfortunately, it's not available in pharmacies, and it's not covered by insurance. But we'll get you as much as we can."

"What happens when I run out?"

"We'll try to buy some for you if you like, but it's pretty expensive." *Something else to look forward to.*

"Your salivary glands have pretty much stopped working due to radiation, so your mouth is very dry. For that you can use Biotene over the counter. There are rinses and toothpaste. There's also a lozenge called XyliMelt. Dry mouth is unpleasant, but it's also bad for your teeth. So you want to treat that too."

I turned a page on my notepad and caught up on what I'd been told.

"As a last resort, we have something we call a 'stomatitis cocktail' for mouth pain. It's also called Magic Mouthwash. We can call in a prescription for the hospital pharmacy to mix for you. It has lidocaine, a local anesthetic, Benadryl for pain, and Maalox to coat your mouth. Let me know if you want to try it."

He excused himself and left the room, returning a few minutes later with three bottles of MuGard, enough for at least a month. I wanted to hug him. I wanted to hug him even more later after I called the pharmaceutical company and found out I would have to pay over $600 a bottle if I ran out.

Trial and error got me through the next couple of weeks. I found that the salt rinses did not help immediately, but after using them persistently for three days the secretions did thin. It became easier to eat and decreased the nausea the secretions caused. I tried Robitussin, but the syrup burned my mouth so badly I had to stop using it.

The effectiveness of the MuGard remained questionable. I do think it helped minimize the sores since they didn't intensify. Robbie told me that, based on other patients with similar complaints, if I hadn't used MuGard my sores and secretions would have been much worse. I didn't notice much change in the dryness in my mouth with Biotene either. But once again, it's likely I would have been much more uncomfortable without it.

Before the remedies above kicked in, I asked for and tried the Magic Mouthwash cocktail. I thought the burning sensation the rinse caused was worse than the pain I already had in my mouth. The burning didn't get better after using it for a few days, so I preferred to use the more conservative methods.

I believe my symptoms were less than usual because I made the effort to follow the regime I'd been given. All in all, the use of these methods did make me more comfortable and my life more tolerable. After trial and error, I was able to find a pattern that improved my symptoms to some extent.

There were some days when my throat pain felt really bad, but not much worse than the sharp pain one gets with a bad cold.

At each appointment, my doctors asked me to rate my pain level on a scale of one to ten. The question didn't always make sense to me. The answer depended on where the pain was and relative to what. But I guess some sort of numerical value helped guide their advice. I reached a level of six or seven, but part of the day I was below that. I took pain meds, but only as mentioned earlier, Tylenol at seven in the morning and two in the afternoon, and Norco at bedtime.

The pain from radiation burns was worse, especially when I touched the area or it was irritated by clothing, and the itching was constant. I avoided touching the burns, kept my skin well moisturized, and wore soft fabrics with open necklines. Most of the time I managed to keep the discomfort tolerable.

In bed at night, I tried to swallow as infrequently as possible and arranged my body such that the sensitive areas of my hands, feet, or radiation burns weren't touching the bedding. It was hard to find the right position, which seemed to change from day to day, but with the pain pill I was taking at bedtime, I usually slept well.

I had mild laryngitis and hoarseness from about week three of radiation therapy that continued well into recovery.

There were times I had disturbing symptoms like a skipped heartbeat or jabbing pain somewhere. I told myself these symptoms weren't related to my cancer treatment. I intentionally and quickly put them out of my mind. I wouldn't allow anxiety to kick in over imaginary problems. I couldn't believe God would give me another problem on top of the cancer to deal with, especially with all my prayers and those who were praying for me. Whatever the reason, all my other health conditions stayed under control.

During the month of February, I sent out four weekly blog posts. I had started writing the blog in hopes that reading about my experiences would be helpful to others, but I came to realize that putting my journey into words caused me to relive the experience, but at the same time I separated my side effects and other medical worries from my wildly-swinging emotions. Instead of having a pity party, I looked for descriptions and explanations of what happened along the way. Also, the many responses I got from fans were heartwarming, encouraging, and touching. Readers told me they were forwarding my blog to friends with cancer and expressed appreciation for sharing my knowledge. The benefits people were getting from my writing eventually led to the writing of this memoir.

I added Paul and Vani, my radiation therapists, to my blog subscriber list. They told me they appreciated knowing what their patients were thinking while they were receiving treatment.

I was happy to know that sharing my story served the purpose for which I wrote it. It's easy to lose a sense of personal worthiness during cancer treatment. A person feels like a burden, dependent on others, at such times. Being able to help others replaces a feeling of uselessness with one of pride and accomplishment.

At the beginning of February, my second month of cancer treatment, I was resigned to the fact that the coming month would be harder than I had at first believed. I had faith, though, that somehow I would get through it. I realized that as I experienced each new side effect, at first it seemed awful. As February wore on, I learned to deal with each new problem. Then, with so many things happening at once, each *individual* problem seemed to fade to a lower level of "awfulness," although my overall condition was going downhill.

Two weeks into the second month of therapy, with two weeks of radiation to go, radiation burns had become life-changing. I was tired all the time and was barely able to function for three hours a day, the time I spent on radiation treatments.

"I'm doing all the things you told me, everything I can, but nothing seems to help. It's so frustrating!" I complained to Dr. Gold.

"Do you think you're becoming depressed? That is very common. Don't demand too much of yourself," he said.

I thought I'd always had a good handle on my emotions. But my face must have indicated otherwise.

"Would you like to see a psychiatrist?"

His question brought me up short. Me? Need a psychiatrist? I remembered how my father, living on a ventilator, became furious at the implication that he wasn't in control of himself and refused to be polite to the staff psychiatrist. I tried to be open-minded about the suggestion I might need help, but I was nearing the end of treatment and I thought I could make it on my own.

By the end of February, I admitted to myself that treating cancer was not for sissies. There were surprises. Treating cancer was harder than I had bargained for. I worried about how much worse I would get, but I still did what I was told. Sometimes I was disappointed, sometimes worried, but not discouraged, despite the significant pain I had by the end of the month. The importance of everything I did was colored by the fear that if I didn't cooperate sufficiently and stay encouraged, the treatment might fail and I might die. And by the realization that even if I did everything I could, the treatment could still fail.

I longed for the experience to be over.

And what I wouldn't have given for a hot shower!

CHAPTER 34
More About Side Effects

"It seemed that you handled the whole experience well. Some people can shut down, but you didn't do that." - John, son

"We were surprised that they didn't place a feeding tube. It was great that you didn't have to have that placed. It would have been something extra to manage and eventually remove, and you probably would have been more depressed by the constant reminder of a tube that you had to service every day." - Bob, son

"I learned some things like what you'd eat or what you tried, like putting butter and honey in oatmeal. I got conscious of some side effects from what you told me and started thinking about telling my new patients or asking them more questions or giving them more choices." - Dolly, daughter-in-law

I shuffled into the kitchen in pajamas and robe about eight one morning, dragging myself from bed later than what I'd done before I started treatment. Chris was sitting in his recliner in our adjacent family room, where I usually found him when he wasn't otherwise occupied. "How are you doing this morning, hon?" he asked, without looking up from the newspaper he was reading.

"About the same," I rasped. Even to my own ears, my reply was unintelligible.

"Huh?" He lifted his head and blinked.

I pointed to my throat, frowned at him, and shook my head. I could hardly get out more than a whisper, but this hoarseness would get better after I ate breakfast and used my voice for a while.

Why doesn't he know by now that I can't talk when I first get up? I've been this way for weeks, I thought. Immediately I felt ashamed. He was being kind and I was taking my frustrations out on him. That wasn't fair.

I can't let this thing get to me! I walked to where he was sitting and dropped a kiss on top of his bald head. He squeezed my arm. I went back into the kitchen to silently prepare the oatmeal that was practically my whole diet now.

Later that morning, Chris walked by the open bathroom doorway and saw me doing the first round of what I called my "dizzy exercises." I was tossing my head rapidly from side to side, like shaking my head "no" vigorously, while fixing my gaze on a spot on the wall.

"No, no, no, no, no," Chris said, singing the words. "I'm surprised this doesn't bring on dizziness instead of preventing it."

Too busy counting the head tosses, I didn't answer him. Then I stood still for a moment to let the room stop moving.

"It does work, number one. And number two, it's actually more effective and less trouble than the exercises I do lying on the bed."

He came to me, drew me into a hug. "I'm glad it works. You don't need another complication."

A few years before I was diagnosed with cancer, I had spells of dizziness, lightheadedness, and bouts of vertigo. After a severe bout of vertigo that kept me in bed for days, a few sessions of physical therapy taught me a series of exercises to reduce the symptoms. Once the severe symptoms cleared up, I tended to be lackadaisical about these exercises. Now I was worried my vertigo would escalate during therapy and took steps to prevent it. I restarted my head-tossing before therapy began, doing the routine for a minute at least twice a day, more often if I had any dizziness.

I drank plenty of water to prevent dehydration and avoided sudden movements. These measures seemed to help. Except for times when I was unusually tired, my dizziness remained under control through therapy and recovery.

My typical day was dramatically changed as a cancer patient.

Most of the side effects I experienced during my two months of therapy involved my mouth and my skin. Other side effects were for the most part minor, but I'm mentioning them because I was constantly aware of them as a possibility and because not everyone's experience with tongue cancer is the same.

Chemotherapy causes changes in the components of the blood in many patients, the most common being anemia and lowering of magnesium, either of which could drop to dangerous levels. For this reason, before each and every infusion of Cetuximab my blood was tested to monitor the effects of therapy on my general health. This included a blood count to detect anemia and a comprehensive metabolic panel to show potential problems involving electrolytes, glucose, liver, kidneys, and more. These are the same basic tests I had as a healthy patient with my yearly general checkup. If these tests were abnormal, changes would have been made to my infusion to correct the condition. My tests stayed basically normal throughout the course. I didn't have to get a transfusion or deal with liver, kidney, diabetes, or other problems that can occur.

My magnesium level was also monitored before every infusion. Up to half of patients treated with Cetuximab experience low magnesium. Magnesium is necessary for healthy heart, muscles, bones, and nerves. It controls energy, blood pressure, blood sugar, and other body functions. My magnesium level never got low. If it had, I would have needed an infusion of magnesium prior to receiving Cetuximab, since it takes too long to build up magnesium with oral medication.

I suspect almost every person undergoing chemotherapy will have some bowel habit changes. I didn't escape that problem, and, in fact, bouts of constipation or diarrhea began with my first infusion. Each person will need to find what works best for them by trial and error and consulting with their oncologist.

My constipation may have been from the pain pills or nausea pills I took, or because I was eating very little food at that time. It was probably a combination. I realized that bowel problems were going to be with me throughout my therapy and took steps right away, so the symptoms didn't get serious.

After eating prunes and drinking prune juice daily resulted in diarrhea, I tried a stool softener called Miralax, which is available over the counter.

Miralax is not a laxative but adds bulk to the stool to make it easier to pass. Mixed with a full glass of water, it tasted a little unpleasant but not bad, and soon I lost my sense of taste anyway. A full dose caused diarrhea again, so I reduced the dose and got my diarrhea under control. I tried taking Miralax on alternate days, but eventually I found that what worked best for me was a half dose taken with dinner every day. I did that throughout therapy and recovery and had no further bowel problems.

Dental problems were a serious concern, but more so after therapy than during it. Radiation to the tongue cannot be delivered without affecting the salivary glands. Just about all patients who have radiation to the neck will have reduced amounts of saliva. After a few weeks of radiation, what little saliva I had was very thick, and my mouth was very dry.

Not only was this a problem from a comfort and ability to eat or speak standpoint, but without the enzymes in saliva, I was likely to develop tooth decay. I used a fluoride rinse through most of my therapy and recovery, stopping only for a few weeks in the middle of therapy when my mouth symptoms were too severe to tolerate the rinse.

I saw my dentist for clearance before I started therapy, but I couldn't see him—unless in case of emergency—during treatment. Because of mucositis, dental work—even cleanings—can cause additional problems, such as infection. But my doctors had stressed that dental care was very important throughout therapy. I flossed, brushed, and used a Waterpik after eating anything—not only meals—and I used a variety of rinses throughout the day for various purposes. In years to come, I could expect tooth decay, tooth loss, and possible bone loss in my jaw.

I didn't have any dental problems during therapy.

My medical team had impressed upon me that my body was undergoing an onslaught by the cancer as well as by the treatment, so I didn't expect to feel generally well. But throughout therapy, although there were unpleasant surprises, I didn't feel as bad as I expected.

I tried to keep up my regular activities, but I rested when I got tired, as I'd been advised. Before therapy began and for the first month, I walked daily for about a mile and a quarter. I needed to stop walking when my energy level got worse and I developed cracks in the skin of my feet and heels from Cetuximab. It became too painful to walk in shoes with backs. Children seem to be able to somehow run in flip-flops, but for me to walk a track in open-back shoes was an invitation to disaster!

I live in a two-story house, and my energy level never got bad enough that stairs became a problem. In fact, I found that when I sat for extended periods or napped, I felt worse afterward, so I tried to stay at least minimally active most of the day. By late afternoon, rather than fatigue I felt generally unwell, my throat pain increased, and I got a little nauseous. That was my signal to tone down my activity. I would read, watch television, and complete my daily health-maintenance schedule. I usually stayed awake until ten or eleven in the evening, sometimes taking a nap in my chair, then regretting it when I woke up feeling bad.

My guess is that, as with the many changes I was undergoing, this general "not-well" sensation was a changed way of feeling fatigue.

Chemotherapy causes hair loss for most patients. Cetuximab, however, doesn't cause as much hair loss as other agents. I had only minor hair loss at my hairlines. I didn't have bald patches, but the hair broke off, leaving bands of slightly reddish scalp with hair about a half inch long on my forehead and at the back of my neck. I don't think this was noticed by anyone but me.

Sometimes I amused myself by wondering what sort of wig I would wear if I did lose my hair. Something long…or loose on my shoulders? I usually didn't like hair on my forehead, but wondered about wearing a wig with bangs. Would I want something natural in my normal color—gray! Or try out being a blond, a redhead, or a brunette. I'd never been a brunette—that could be fun.

Although I didn't go bald, my hair grew slowly for more than six months. All my body hair got coarse and brittle, especially my eyebrows. On the other hand, my eyelids looked bald, and I had thinning hair on my legs and armpits.

I didn't attempt to shave during therapy and recovery, as I'd been warned that shaving could be irritating. My skin was dry and leathery (snakeskin!) and cut easily. I learned to be careful when making fists or other movements of my fingers or toes to avoid cutting my skin with my own nails.

Chemotherapy agents can cause some hearing loss, either temporary or permanent. Cetuximab usually doesn't do this, but the radiation field for my therapy included my ears. My hearing was good, and I didn't notice any hearing loss throughout treatment nor during recovery.

Some people have allergic or other adverse reactions to chemotherapy that would usually occur while the infusion was in progress. For this reason, Benadryl is often given as a premedication before an infusion. Reactions can be severe. I didn't have any reactions, except after the first infusion when I had nausea and muscle weakness hours later. For the rest of my infusions, I was given additional injections through my intravenous line prior to my infusion to prevent nausea. The precaution worked. The only effects I had thereafter were slight lightheadedness and fatigue immediately after the infusion.

I'm delighted to be able to say I never vomited during or after treatment! This had been one of my biggest fears about chemotherapy. Except for the reaction to my first infusion, I had nausea to some extent almost every day, but the feeling was moderate and controlled by the oral medication I was given, which I took only when I needed it. I rarely took more than one pill a day, and some days my nausea was so mild or transitory I didn't need medication.

Fortunately, pain was not a significant factor for me either. I suspect I tolerate pain more easily and minimize its effects more than most people. I had always been one to push through pain as far as possible, to work on days most people would stay in bed, to be stoic. I thought of myself as "Polish woman, strong as bull!" Most of the time I was proud of myself, but I must admit that showing strength lowers the sympathy level and creates expectations in the minds of others that are sometimes hard to meet.

That does *not* mean I didn't have pain, but that it took a higher level to put me out of commission. Since the effects of radiation are cumulative, the worst pain I experienced was from radiation burns, not during therapy but in the recovery period. Not everyone has the same level of tolerance and determination. For some dealing with side effects will be harder than it was for me. Others will find it easier.

Before the radiation burns developed, I usually had some level of pain, but not enough to interfere significantly with activities. When my pain level increased, I controlled it with Tylenol and Norco and was able to sleep well most nights.

My oncologist felt my back and abdomen for tenderness at each visit. Some people have stomach pain, but I didn't. I imagine this could be a problem for those who have not managed constipation and diarrhea well, who are eating the wrong foods, or who have reactions that involve their liver. I didn't have any of that.

Dr. Gold had reminded me that the GI tract is lined with tissue susceptible to mucositis.

"Mucositis is one of the hardest things you'll experience during your treatment," he said, his eyes soft with sympathy. "It can affect not only your mouth, but your throat and your esophagus. And it can last three months after you finish radiation. There is little we can do for it."

I did get some chest discomfort from time to time after eating. I attributed that to heartburn, likely related to mucositis moving down my esophagus. The upper esophagus was also in my radiation field. For me, this pain was rare and mild.

I occasionally had a mild headache of short duration—under an hour. I didn't experience any other pain.

I lost my appetite, had difficulty eating and swallowing.

I was seventy-five years old when I was diagnosed with cancer, and I didn't get to that age without some health issues unrelated to cancer. I was concerned that those other conditions might get out of control when my body was subjected to the rigors of cancer treatment. That didn't happen.

I was careful to avoid catching an infection. I stayed home as much as possible and washed my hands almost compulsively. I feared my blood pressure would soar, but it was measured regularly, stayed normal, and I never had to change my prior medications. I stopped taking the prescription I had been given for anxiety after the first few days of treatment.

I reminded myself that my treatment plan for tongue cancer had a high success rate, but that the treatment itself would be tough.

It was tough. But then, most people have experienced tough spells from other diseases, burns, or accidents at some time in their life. But it bears repeating that there is a major difference when facing cancer because so many problems are happening at the same time and one has to live with the problems for a long time before they get better.

I've included this information so that other tongue cancer patients and those who care for them will know that there are conditions I didn't mention while detailing my experience, because I didn't experience them.

I feel strongly that my positive attitude and cooperation with the program defined by my doctors in addition to the research protocol I was enrolled in helped to make the treatment easier for me. I hope others will either benefit from my experience or have the strength to develop their own ways of coping with cancer. I believe I would have felt worse were it not for my cooperation. This belief inspired me when things got tough. I felt I was personally important for the success of my treatment.

CHAPTER 35
Life Before Cancer: Retirement and Chorus, 2008

Life seemed pretty good after I retired in early 2008. Chris retired the following year.

Shortly after retiring I accepted a position as Vice President of Development for the Downers Grove Choral Society. Joining the chorus had made a real change in my life.

The music! It was glorious, in a way I had never experienced. It filled my heart with joy and moved me to tears. We gave three concerts a year, and for each we hired a professional orchestra and professional soloists to perform works of the greatest masters of classical music. The addition of professionals allowed the chorus the opportunity to elevate the performance.

I wanted to support the group any way I could, but at first, I had no idea the magnitude of the commitment development requires. I had to write numerous grant requests every year, run fundraising events, and network with local businesses and organizations to obtain support for the group. I did a good job, and I enjoyed the work, but it took a lot of time.

The hard work had many rewards. One of the most memorable was the week I spent working closely with Metropolitan Opera star, baritone Sherrill Milnes. During all the planning and rehearsals for the two performances of Elijah we did, he learned that I was the person who best responded to his requests, not just willingly and efficiently, but because I enjoyed being his go-to person. We fell into chatting and joking during downtime and formed a friendship that lasted a few years—until time and distance took its toll.

But there was another question I had to get out of my system. As many had suggested, I wondered if I had what it took to be a writer. I joined a writer's group in 2009 to find out.

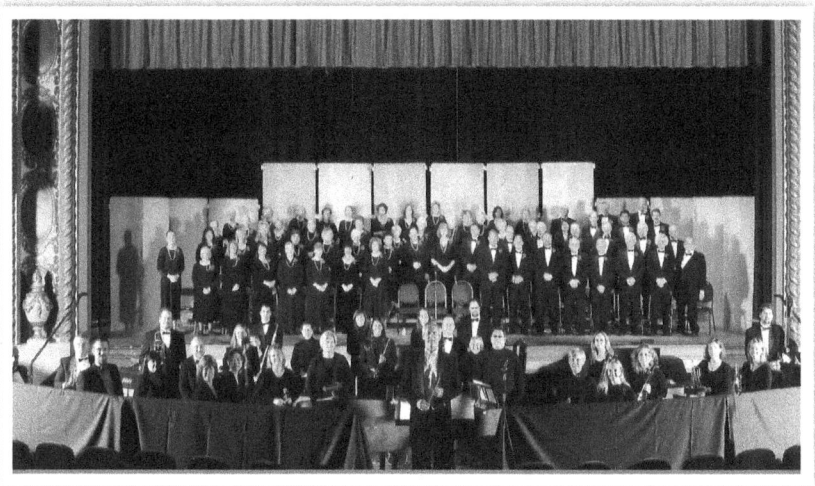

Downers Grove Choral Society in Concert, Tivoli Theater

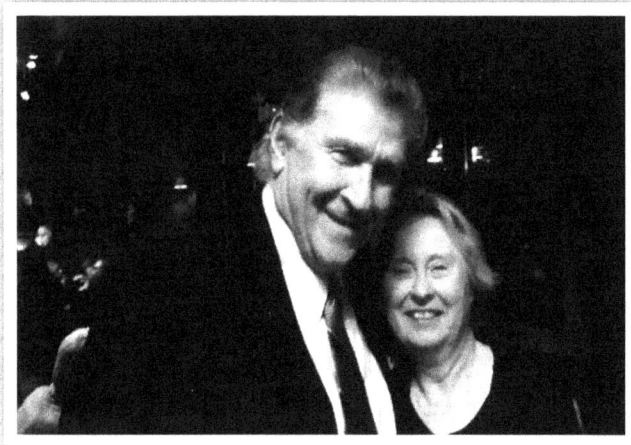

Me after concert with Metropolitan Opera Star Sherrill Milnes

CHAPTER 36
Support Services: Nutrition

"You have to breathe, you have to eat, you have to swallow, and you don't think about these things because you take it for granted. When I brush my teeth, when I eat, this is going to hurt, it tastes bad." - Dolly, daughter-in-law

Even before I started treatment for cancer, I had lost five pounds. It was not from the disease, and not from the therapy, but from worry. Unlike people who binge-eat when nervous, all my life I lost my appetite when I was anxious. I had battled with my weight for most of my life, and at the time of my diagnosis I was nearing a hundred and seventy pounds, the most I'd ever weighed, and much too much for my five-foot three-inch height. The thought that I would be likely to lose weight during my treatment seemed like a silver lining to me. If I had to go through a nasty time, at least I could come out of the experience with a new slender body.

That wasn't how my oncologists saw it. They insisted it was important to the success of my treatment to maintain my current weight. Goodbye silver lining.

I lost another five pounds in the first week of treatment due to throat pain from my biopsy and nausea and constipation after my first chemotherapy infusion. This brought me to ten pounds less than my pre-cancer weight. My medical team was not happy. I promised them I would do better, motivated by my strong fear of having a feeding tube.

After two weeks of radiation therapy my anxiety and constipation were over, but side effects were developing that made it hard to eat. I had mild nausea. It was painful and difficult to swallow. My taste buds were acting wacky, and I had sores in my mouth.

Soon, not only did I suffer from loss of appetite due to anxiety, but everything I put in my mouth either tasted lousy or had no taste. My brain had me thinking I'd really enjoy the milkshake I planned for lunch, but my body told me I just wasn't hungry. I tolerated most foods well enough at that time, but I had to force myself to eat. Each successive mouthful became harder and harder to swallow. My appetite wasn't poor, it was nonexistent.

At my second chemotherapy infusion I saw a dietitian. This wasn't my idea. It was prescribed by my oncologists, part of the standard treatment plan.

"During cancer treatment is the worst time to lose weight—the body needs nutrition to fight the disease as well as to deal with the treatment you're getting," my dietitian explained. "During treatment you should expect to burn calories up to three times faster than normal. You have to give your body the tools it needs."

I hadn't thought of that. In essence my body was using calories: one, for its normal daily functions; two, to fight cancer; and three, to rebuild the cells that cancer treatment destroyed. I needed triple the amount of energy I would require when healthy.

My dietitian urged me to maintain a high calorie count. The reasons she gave for this were convincing. If I lost weight too quickly, I would lose muscle mass. Muscles are important—my heart, for instance, is composed of muscle. Heart disease, with its potential for sudden death, frightened me even more than cancer.

Poor nutrition would also interfere with my body's immune system and its ability to fight cancer. My doctors had explained that it was my immune system that actually killed my cancer cells after they were tagged by Cetuximab. I had to keep my immune system healthy since it was at least an equal component to the action of chemotherapy. There was even a danger if I lost too much weight that my radiation mask would no longer fit snugly and keep me immobile during radiation therapy!

I had to adjust my normal eating habits, which I knew were rather sloppy.

A lifelong yoyo dieter, I had gained and lost the same twenty pounds or so every eight or ten years throughout my life, and with each cycle I retained a bit more weight. I had fooled my metabolism into thinking I could exist on 800 calories a day without dropping a pound. I already routinely avoided fats and carbs, had done so for years, and was only able to maintain, not lose, weight at that calorie level.

Now I was told:
- Eat as many calories as possible.
- Add butter, sugar, cream to everything. The more the better.
- High calorie, high protein is your goal.
- Drink milkshakes and smoothies, eat pudding and ice cream.

That may sound like a dream come true, but after so many years of battling weight in the only way that seemed to work for me, in my guilty mind I was eating *bad* foods. This seemed equivalent to me as if I grew up a child of the Depression and was told it was okay to buy anything I wanted, squander all my savings on trivia, and let food and possessions go to waste. Oh, yeah. That's right. My parents lived through the Depression and transferred that guilt to me too. Eating the foods my nutritionist recommended increased my anxiety.

Despite loss of appetite, inability to eat, and guilt, I had to get good nutrition if my treatment was going to be a success. Plus I couldn't forget my fear of the feeding tube.

To be sure I understood and kept the right attitude about nutrition, dietitians saw me every Monday after my radiation therapy.

I usually saw student dietitians first and then the staff dietitian assigned to my case would finish the visit. The students mostly came in pairs. They were knowledgeable and enthusiastic, different young women each visit. It was clear that they all wanted me to succeed and took a personal interest in my care. They tag-teamed each other, reviewed what I was eating, asked about any difficulties I might be having, checked my weight, and offered suggestions. They set a calorie level for me—1500 to 1800 calories per day. Since I generally ate less than 1000 calories when I was well, I thought that was too much, but said I'd try.

I enjoyed talking to the students, feeling a little like a teacher that was helping them learn their subject. They looked at each other, grinning with satisfaction when I agreed with them. They listened when I disagreed. They took notes on what I said. Our conversations were lighthearted, with smiles and laughs. After the students, the registered dietitian came in to review my progress and the students' advice and summarized each session.

I told the students: "Pain isn't much of a problem for me. Nausea and taste are a bigger deal. Everything tastes awful, salty or metallic, and I have no appetite. A few bites and I feel full and don't want to eat anymore. If I push it, I get sick to my stomach. Imagine you're already stuffed, and someone puts a full plate of food you hate in front of you and tells you to eat it all. Or try to eat a large quantity of rich food when you're feeling sick to your stomach. That's what it's like."

"Do you throw up?"

"No, but again, try to make yourself eat when everything you put in your mouth makes you feel sick."

"You need to get more calories into smaller portions of food then. That's why Ensure is good, and high-calorie additions," the students said.

I could just drink Ensure and call it done, I thought. But I was afraid if I stopped chewing and swallowing, I would end up with that feeding tube, and if I didn't eat solid food my constipation would recur.

They had me step on a scale and recorded my weight in my chart weekly, comparing it to the previous week and my pre-treatment weight. I showed them my journal.

"You are actually doing quite well. Even on a lower calorie count than recommended, you've gained back a couple of the pounds you lost." Both students looked surprised.

I was advised to eat smaller meals, but six meals a day. Not only would I have to confront my absence of appetite six times but also prepare meals and clean up that many times. In addition, I had the onerous dental hygiene routine every time I ate.

My dietitian gave me handouts with suggestions for high-calorie foods to pick from. The lists included things I could add to my food, like butter and honey, to provide more calories. They gave me suggested menus. They encouraged me to drink Ensure or similar products to keep my calorie level up. They gave me samples of nutrition drinks. In my daily journal, I already recorded my calorie count, how I felt, and problems and successes. I recorded my weight weekly.

I gave up the idea of eating the foods I was accustomed to and ate for survival instead of pleasure. Every time I sat down to eat it was an effort. I would start the meal with a good attitude, determined to accomplish my calorie goal for the day. I would look at the food in front of me, which was unappealing, no matter that I had prepared my favorite foods in an attempt to enjoy them. I'd put a small portion in my mouth and chew it, working it into a ball. All my efforts were in vain. I wanted to spit the food out of my mouth, but I'd force myself to swallow it. Then I'd control a wave of nausea and wait for the disgusting feeling to pass before trying another bite.

"How's your sense of smell?" my dietitian asked.

"No change in that," I replied.

"That's good. Some patients lose their sense of smell too."

"I'm not so sure it's good. Sometimes cooking odors make me sick. When you're not hungry at all, smelling food isn't a good thing. It's almost as bad as trying to eat."

"Well, you'll appreciate your sense of smell better once this is all over."

Although my attitude was positive and I saw the sense in what I was being asked to do, when added to other recommendations from my specialists, I reminded myself again that staying alive was now a full-time job. The day simply wasn't long enough to do everything. I had to decide the most effective advice, follow that, and hope for the best.

In addition, I was spending midday Monday through Friday at the hospital, so my food had to be portable to eat in the car or between appointments.

I discovered that packaged biscuits and rolls from the dairy case, the ones that come in a tube that you take home and bake, are small and high in calories. I made a sandwich from them with peanut butter, jelly, and cheese. Lunch came to 380 calories, and it was portable. I felt proud of this discovery for a week or two, until I couldn't handle bread anymore. It turned into a thick tasteless blob in my mouth that I couldn't swallow without wanting to vomit.

After that, I traveled with little containers of hardboiled eggs, cottage cheese, and pudding. Soon even the eggs and cottage cheese were difficult. Almost all food tasted really bad.

"What are you eating now that you *can* tolerate?" my dietitian asked.

"I can always eat oatmeal and drink Ensure. Other foods are iffy," I said.

"Then eat oatmeal and Ensure," I was told.

"We may have some Ensure samples. What flavor do you like?"

"Anything. It doesn't make any difference. Everything tastes the same."

I told her I added cinnamon sugar, butter, and cream to oatmeal to bulk up calories, and a cup of coffee with cream—my only coffee of the day, since caffeine is discouraged. Thus prepared, breakfast was 250 calories. Ensure was 350. So, with these two things alone I was almost halfway to my calorie count.

On another visit I felt discouraged. "I do okay earlier in the day, but by afternoon or evening it's really hard to eat anything at all."

"That's because side effects build during the day. Take advantage and load yourself up early in the day so you can eat less in the evening."

A few of their suggestions didn't work for me. Some people like cold foods like ice cream and milkshakes. I found warm foods easier to swallow, even warm water. Ice cream, no matter what flavor, tasted like salty metal to me. I also couldn't tolerate sugarless candy or gum. These burned and then left an unpleasant, sickening taste in my mouth, sometimes for hours afterward. To keep my mouth "busy" I preferred warm—never hot!—water or tea.

In addition to these measures, I found the following tips to be helpful:
- Avoid foods that are spicy or acidic.
- Avoid alcoholic beverages and mouthwashes.
- Minimize caffeine. I limited coffee to one cup in the morning and added cream instead of drinking it black to reduce acidity.
- Identify the convenient foods you can eat without difficulty and keep eating them.
- Don't try to force foods that aren't working when something else will work.
- If oatmeal and Ensure are all you can eat, then eat oatmeal and Ensure.
- Mix sips of water with food when the mouth is dry or when you are having trouble swallowing. But don't try to swallow foods of different consistency (liquid, solid, dry, etc.) at the same time. To avoid this, drop your chin to your chest and mix the food in your mouth with water before trying to swallow. There is more space in this part of the mouth.
- Swallowing may be more difficult. Sometimes it feels like a lump in

the throat that doesn't want to go down. Be patient. It will.
- Swallow consciously, with care and attention. If coughing or sticking of food occurs, stop until it's controlled, then try again. I had little coughing and minimal sticking but stayed very aware.
- I found that foods that were slightly warm were best for me. Some people like cold foods, especially milkshakes, but I couldn't tolerate ice cream.
- Experiment but avoid hot foods like the plague.
- It may be helpful to sip something like warm tea.

My reward? After my initial weight loss prior to treatment, over two months of cancer treatment I lost only ten more pounds! My medical team was happy with that result. I felt some pride in my success and their pleasure, but I couldn't help but feel a little gypped. I had wanted that svelte new body.

CHAPTER 37
Support Services: Speech Therapy

"The amount of coughing seemed tough. Sometimes it seemed that you wouldn't make it through the spell, and you had a hard time breathing. Those episodes seemed scary. I wasn't expecting radiation to do that much damage. That surprised me." - John, son

My mother was still living in her home in 2010 but spent weekends with Chris and me. We were having hot dogs for lunch at the kitchen table, Mom sat in her customary chair with her back to the window so she had good light to read, and I sat across from her. We were both reading, until I heard sounds of distress.

I looked up to see Mom clutching at the table to keep from falling, each breath a wheezing effort that stopped midway, her eyes bulging. I realized immediately that she was choking. I ran for help to Amy, my neighbor next door who was a nurse, while Chris stayed with Mom and dialed 911 for assistance.

Amy rushed in, took one look, stepped behind Mom, pulled her upright, wrapped her arms around Mom with her fist below Mom's ribs, and began to press against Mom's diaphragm rhythmically. Amy uttered, "Come on, come on, come on," with each forceful thrust. It seemed to take forever. Mom just didn't seem ready to give up that chunk of hot dog. But eventually it came out.

By the time the ambulance arrived, Amy had eased Mom back down into her chair and Mom was breathing deeply but unobstructed. We all thought it was a good idea to allow the paramedics to take Mom to the hospital to be checked, and Mom agreed.

During a three-day stay, the hospital determined that Mom was no longer swallowing properly. Her food was aspirating into her windpipe instead of being routed to her esophagus.

At the base of the tongue, the esophagus (which connects the mouth to the stomach) and the trachea (the airway that connects to the lungs) are next to each other in the space called the pharynx. There's a little valve at the base of the pharynx, the epiglottis, that closes when we swallow to keep food from going down the windpipe and into the lungs. Mom's epiglottis was no longer working properly. This happens with the elderly, but in Mom's case it was likely to be a late effect of the stroke she had had some years before this incident.

The end result was that Mom could no longer take food by mouth. A tube was inserted in her abdomen, called a gastrostomy. She was fed by attaching a syringe filled with a liquid formula to the gastrostomy, then pushing the feeding directly into her stomach. She did well on the tube for years and otherwise led a normal life, although she could no longer live alone, so she moved in with us. And, of course, the pleasures of eating were lost to her.

When the possibility of my needing to have a feeding tube was mentioned, the vision of Mom struggling to breathe came back to me over and over. And, of course, I had intimate knowledge of what it was like to live with a gastrostomy.

I knew, for instance, that although the liquid went directly to Mom's stomach, some taste would back up into her mouth, and it was a taste Mom didn't like. I already had significant nausea. I feared, correctly, that if I vomited from the taste of the feeding I could aspirate. I knew what it was like to have to keep the wound clean. I knew how Mom longed for the pleasures of eating, and that the sprays available to give her the sensation of taste didn't do the trick, so she soon discontinued them.

I didn't want a feeding tube. It wasn't something to fear. I could live with it indefinitely, but I also knew it was unpleasant.

Speech therapists evaluate and advise patients not only about speech, but they also provide training for swallowing disorders. Speech therapy is routine for treatment of tongue cancer, but if it hadn't been I would have asked for it due to my fear of a feeding tube.

Even if I had a tube placed, I knew I would have to be concerned about swallowing, breathing, speaking, and long-term lifestyle. When I pictured the area where I knew my primary cancer was, I would imagine my throat swelling, closing off my airway. I imagined choking, food sticking, being unable to breathe. It hadn't happened, but I needed reassurance over and over.

Judith, a speech therapist, saw me after radiation therapy every Friday. While oncologists were managing treatment, my therapists and my nurses were teaching me how to manage everyday life and how to survive not only my cancer but my treatment and recovery. The primary reason for a tube was to be sure I got sufficient nutrition. Dietitians were helping me with that, but I'd also have to have a tube if I became unable to swallow.

Dr. Fidler's nurse Mary's words when preparing me for my first infusion haunted me: "We can't promise you won't need a feeding tube. It will help if you're religious about mouth care, swallowing exercises, and nutrition. But if you lose too much weight, I'm afraid you'll have to have a tube. Most people are able to get off the tube when they start eating well again." And I remembered the shock I felt when the implication sunk in that some people *don't* get off the tube.

With the dreaded feeding tube hanging over my head, it was very important to me to not lose the ability to swallow. So I welcomed help.

On my first visit with Judith, she asked questions and let me explain my fears.

"Let's see how everything is working now," she said. On a nearby counter was a tray with foods of various thicknesses, including water, applesauce, and graham crackers.

The therapist put her fingers on my throat and left them there while I took a few swallows of each sample.

"Good," she said. "Your swallowing feels normal. Now let's see what we can do to be sure it stays that way."

She then demonstrated a series of exercises. Some were familiar, since I had watched my mother do them. The series took about fifteen minutes, and I was to do it three times a day. The goal was to strengthen and train the muscles involved in the swallowing process.

One of the exercises was to stick my tongue out a little, hold it with my lips or teeth, and swallow. It was awkward at first. In fact, it's still awkward. Try it and you'll see what I mean.

Another was to sing the vowel "E," starting low, going very high (falsetto), sustaining at the high pitch, then dropping to very low. That was easier to do, but embarrassing if doing it in public, and I spent much of my day at the hospital.

A third was to "dry swallow," without food, forcefully. That was surprisingly difficult to do. Normal swallowing was easy so far, but engaging all the neck muscles with no food felt unnatural and I never felt like I was doing it right.

"The best exercise of all is actually swallowing your food," she said.

I'm not proud of my compliance with these exercises. Despite my motivation, I sometimes forgot to do them, sometimes I was too tired, and sometimes it just didn't work out. I tried to do the routines in the car to and from hospital visits or whenever I remembered during the day, or to do the less "obvious" exercises in public during wait times. I got some exercises done every day, and my therapist was happy. She could see I was doing well and was more compliant than the average patient.

I brought a list of questions to each visit. Being careful not to make promises—medicine is not an exact science—Judith nonetheless set my mind at rest about my image of my throat swelling to the point of closing.

"Your ENT is the best person to discuss that. However, I can tell you that is *not* something we expect to happen."

"Then why do many people with this diagnosis get feeding tubes?"

"Some aren't as cooperative as you. Some can't eat due to pain, not due to ability to swallow. Your swallowing muscles will always work. However, side effects limit how *effective* the process is. You can minimize the side effects by doing the exercises, whether you're having problems or not."

She told me what to watch for: coughing, sticking of food that was not cleared by multiple swallows, and congestion after meals.

Despite the exercises, side effects did change the way I swallowed food, partly because of pain when swallowing and partly because radiation to the area seemed to make it harder to do. Swallowing became, of necessity, a conscious thing. If I swallowed too quickly or if food hit my soft palate or the back of my throat unexpectedly, food stuck or I had a coughing spell.

I didn't gag, but sometimes I could feel the food staying at the top of my esophagus. In that case I'd have to wait for it to move down. Other times I would have to force food back into my mouth and swallow it again. Then mucositis developed and caused thick mucus but also sore spots on my tongue, cheeks, and gums, which limited the way I moved food around in my mouth. If the food, or even air, hit the back of my throat, it could trigger a coughing spell that was hard to stop.

Swallowing a number of times continuously, what I called repeat-swallowing, such as one does when chugging a glass of water, was hard to do. I could feel my muscles tensing and I feared choking.

"I put food in my mouth and chew it into a ball, but then I can't swallow it because it's too thick and dry. I add water to thin it out. Sometimes I cough because the water drizzles down while the solid food sticks."

Judith sympathized. "Yes, swallowing different consistencies can be hard. Try this: when you want to mix the foods in your mouth, drop your chin and let the food come to the front of your mouth to mix. There's more room for it there."

That worked like a charm! I also found that it was helpful to swish some water in an empty mouth every now and then and swallow that, so that little particles hiding below my tongue or beside my cheeks didn't surprise me and set me coughing.

Through most of my therapy and recovery, I had a sore throat for at least a part of each day. I usually woke up to find that swallowing was painful. After a few consecutive swallows while eating breakfast, the pain would go away. It got more severe again in the late afternoon and evening, but again got better whenever I was eating. It was especially noticeable in bed at night, but since I swallow so infrequently during the night it didn't interfere with my sleep.

"Some of the pills they're having me take I swear were meant for horses. What do I do if I can't get them down?" I worried. I always managed to swallow pills, but on occasion they did seem to stick for a time at the back of my throat and I had to work them down with water.

"You can crush them or twist the capsules apart. Another thing you can do is put the pill in a spoonful of pudding. It seems to make pills slide down easier." I didn't have to try that, but I hope I remember it!

My reward? The result was that I never had to have the dreaded feeding tube. I was able to eat—and breathe!—throughout therapy and recovery, despite the fact that everything tasted like *&^%$#@. I'm firmly convinced that the exercises and discussions with my speech therapist made life easier for me.

PART THREE

After Treatment

CHAPTER 38
Treatment Ends
March 1, 2018

"When you finish, we celebrate. It is always a relief that you have reached this point, and things will improve. Sometimes patients think they're finished so they will be fine, but it's a long process." - Dolly, daughter-in-law

March 1, 2018. My last radiation treatment. I had my last infusion one week earlier, on February 22. After March 1 I would recover at home. No more radiation, no more infusions, no more daily trips to Rush. Eight infusions, thirty-five radiation treatments, two months of altered life came to a sudden stop.

I had watched other patients reach their last day of radiation therapy. They made the day a big deal. I, too, wanted to do something nice to say goodbye to my radiation team. Chris and I stopped at Dunkin' Donuts and got boxes of muffins, bagels, and donuts for the radiation therapy department. We stopped at the hospital's coffee shop and got gift certificates for the front desk staff, for Robbie, for Vani, and for Paul. I had prepared personal letters of thanks and autographed copies of my books for Dr. Layan and Dr. Gold.

The previous week, we had also brought small gifts for the oncology department the day of my last infusion. That same day I had given the infant cap I knitted to Dr. Fidler for her little boy. She would soon be taking maternity leave.

Most cancer patients are happy and relieved to successfully finish treatment. I was too, but despite my honest wish to express gratitude to those who had treated me, I wasn't in much of a mood for fanfare. For one thing, I was too sick and in too much discomfort.

I didn't feel the customary relief most cancer patients felt knowing they would no longer be bound to a daily treatment schedule. Instead, I felt deserted. I hated goodbyes under any circumstances. In this case, goodbye meant the absence of these people, who had become friends, from my life. They had taught me, supported me, and encouraged me every step of the way. It also meant I no longer had the feeling of safety they gave me. Until they were about to go out of my life, I hadn't realized how important it was that I could rely on seeing them every day.

So, I said my goodbyes, not with joy on my face, but with tears in my eyes. From that day on, if I didn't feel well, I wouldn't have the opportunity to discuss it right away with someone knowledgeable.

It was especially hard to say goodbye to Dr. Gold. I had gotten dependent on his day-to-day presence and gentle reassurance. I hoped he would stay at Rush after he completed his residency, but coincidentally his last day was the same as mine. He would be leaving to begin a fellowship in Massachusetts.

"Remember," he said, "therapy is over, but you still have a way to go. Radiation damage is cumulative. You're going to get worse before you get better. It will be months before you recover to your new normal. Some symptoms may be permanent, but you've done so well I don't expect anything major."

I stood near him, tears in my eyes. "But…you can't leave. I need you."

He gave me a hug then, the hug I'd wanted throughout the last two months. It felt a little stiff, but when I stepped back, I saw that his eyes were shiny too. I hoped he would remember me from the copy of *The Mystery at Black Partridge Woods* that I autographed for him.

Oh, I could ask for an appointment with one of my doctors. I could call Bob or Dolly. If I did either of those things, I had to first decide that what concerned me at that moment was bad enough to consult someone about. What would be the purpose of such a call? Another need for reassurance? I didn't have to make decisions like that when I was in daily contact with people who cared about my comfort, understood and sympathized with my complaints. I could ask and get advice about little things.

I would have routine follow-up appointments with my doctors, nurses, and therapists, but I would never see Vani and Paul, my radiation therapists, nor the fellows and students again. No professionals were taking care of me daily. This left a huge vacuum in my life.

I went home to stay there and let my body fix itself.

And so, on March 2, 2018, I woke up knowing I was on my own now. My medical team had given me their best shot—literally!—and now it was up to my body, my God, and me to make the most of it.

> *Recovery: That's what the medical team called this period of done-but-not-quite-well-yet.*

Recovery (definition): Return to a normal state of health, mind, or strength.

Yes, that's what I wanted all right—nothing exorbitant—just to be normal again. After more than three months I was tired of focusing my mind only on my health and crashing every afternoon. I wanted to be rid of nausea and pain. I wanted my life back. But it was so *)%$^* slow!

I asked myself once again: *When is it my turn?* I wanted to focus on myself—not on my health, but with the freedom and ability to do the things I had always wanted to do but had to put off due to responsibilities I couldn't ignore. I wanted to spend more time with my family, traveling, reading, and writing more books.

My doctors said I was progressing more rapidly than most patients, but not to expect overnight recovery. Remember, radiation was a cumulative process—it would take a while. Although I was no longer getting radiation treatments, side effects could continue to occur, even months later. My body had undergone a lot of changes already, but there were even more changes to come—some new, some not so bad, some worse than I expected. I would improve, but it would be slow.

I listened to what they said but without much concern. I had done well so far, hadn't I? It had been hard, as they warned, but I had cooperated with my doctors, done my best to do whatever they'd told me to do. In my case, any more side effects would surely be minimal, I reasoned.

I should have known better by then. When Dr. Thomas first told me I had cancer, I tried to deny it to myself. Then I minimized how side effects would change my life. Why should I believe any differently now that I was in the recovery phase? Perhaps underestimating my disease was my way of coping with my desire to be well, when in fact there was still a long way to go.

So, once again, anxious to have my old life back, I convinced myself that recovery would be easy for me.

Like everything I learned about cancer, recovery is difficult but doable.

CHAPTER 39
Life Before Cancer: Retirement, Mom, and Writing, 2008-2012

I *was enjoying retired life, but life changed once again when my mother had a choking spell. At the hospital, it was discovered that, probably as a late effect of her stroke years earlier, she could no longer swallow without some of the food going into her lungs. She had a feeding tube placed, and since she was no longer able to live alone, she moved in with us.*

We had plenty of room for Mom. We gave her two rooms upstairs to use as bedroom and sitting room, along with the hallway bathroom. She had her own television, brought her bedroom set, easy chairs, and whatever personal items she wanted with her. She had access to our entire house during the day. We redecorated her bedroom as she liked, tried to help her find things to occupy her time, and valued her privacy. It wasn't her own home, but she lived comfortably.

When Mom was settled in, I was already sixty-six years old. Writing and publishing took a long time, so I had no time to waste. I didn't spend time writing essays or short stories. I decided to try writing a novel right away. But what would I write?

It had to be a mystery, because I had been reading mysteries since I found Perry Mason paperbacks in our attic when I was in eighth grade. And it had to be set in Lemont, because I loved the town, with its unique scenery. It had to be a historical mystery because of Lemont's quirky yet important history. Ghost stories and other reported paranormal activity in the area also made it possible to indulge my fascination with the unusual.

So, shortly after Mom moved in with us, I began volunteering in the archives at the Lemont Area Historical Society.

"Don't you have enough to do?" Mom asked.

She had a point. Mom, the chorus, the library, and my writing took a lot of time, but I enjoyed all those activities. I'd never been one to take the easy route or to give anything up. The idea was that I would have access to information I might need when writing about Lemont's history.

Mom mostly took care of herself, I rationalized. She only needed oversight and help with feedings and going up and down stairs. I was just committing to the historical society one morning a week.

I began to spend time now and then playing with ideas and typing them into my computer. When I wrote something I liked, I'd read it to Mom. I don't think she ever thought I'd actually finish a novel. She thought my idea of including a ghost in my story was rather silly. When I suggested including an event from her teen years, she shook her head.

"Why would you want to include that? Who would care?"

Much as I loved Mom, and we had a lot in common, things I found memorable and endearing bewildered her. She was a practical woman with little interest in remembering things she viewed as embarrassing moments. She was ashamed of the fact that her father was an immigrant who died from tuberculosis and that she had the same disease when I was a baby. I, on the other hand, found those facts highlighted her personal strengths and character.

Mom had lived to see her grandson John, and his wife Clare, move an hour away to a far western suburb. She saw the birth of two great-grandsons, John's boys Collin and Aidan.

She lived to see her grandson Bob give up his career at Ford in 2003 and enroll in medical school. Bob had become a gastroenterologist and married Dolly, a medical oncologist, in 2011. Bob's career change was a big help to us during my mother's illnesses.

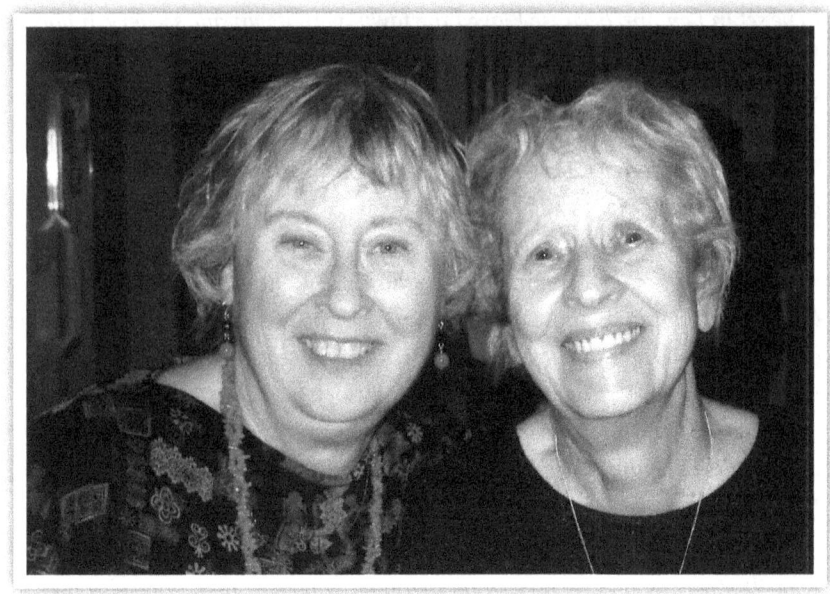

Me and Mom

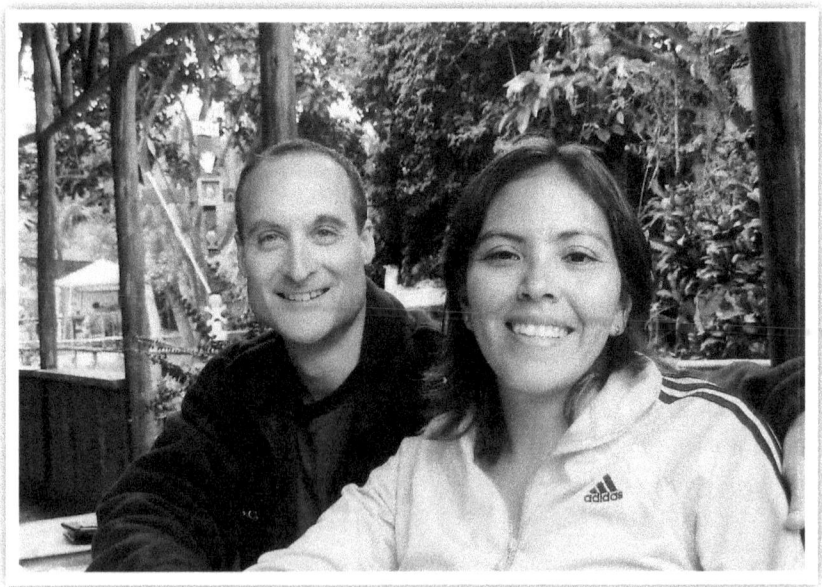

Bob and Dolly

CHAPTER 40
Recovery Begins
March 2018

" You seemed to get things done when you were going through recovery. Some people would just stay home and not do anything." - John, son

"Your blog must have been cathartic for you and helped see you through."
- Bob, son

On my last day of radiation therapy, a week after my last chemotherapy infusion, I had throat pain when I swallowed, no appetite, thick secretions in my mouth, mild nausea with food, and could eat only a limited diet consisting of mainly oatmeal, pudding, and Ensure. My neck was red, blistered, and painful from radiation burns, requiring steroids, lubricants, and soaks. I had a rash from chemotherapy in addition to the radiation burns, my skin was dry and sensitive, and I had painful skin splits on my hands and feet. What little sense of taste I had was out of whack—everything tasted the same, salty, metallic, and bad. Swallowing was an effort and rather tricky. All day I followed a healthcare schedule, leaving little time for personal matters. By mid-afternoon I was exhausted.

During the first week post treatment, there was little improvement. My skin conditions remained the same. My mouth was so dry it was hard to sleep at night. Food seemed to take a while to travel down my esophagus.

I tried to suck on a lemon drop to moisten my mouth, but I got sick to my stomach and had to take a Zofran tablet. Clearly, I wasn't ready to add foods yet. I didn't expect things to change in a week, so I was patient at that point. I told myself I would start feeling better soon, perhaps even the next week.

During that week I received in the mail a little pale blue metal box, painted with tiny green vines and pink flowers, and wrapped with a white lace ribbon. The top read, "Prayer Box." Inside was a tiny block of notepaper two inches by three and a half inches, and a four-inch pencil. The inscription on the inside upper lid read:

> "When your head starts to worry and your mind just can't rest, put your prayers down on paper and let God do the rest!"

On each and every day since I started treatment, my friend Dorothy had said a little prayer for me and written on a page of the notepad. The first day, dated January 10, said:

> "Keep Pat comfortable and safe. Make sure the treatment is correct and works. Support her emotionally and give her my love."

January 13 said, "My dearest friend, I love you. I offer up any pain I experience to alleviate any pain you may have thrust upon you. I don't want you to hurt. I pray for you every day."

February 3 said, "Please don't take my sunshine away." With a little drawing of a smiley face.

February 17 said, "Don't worry, be Patsy." My family called me Snooky when I was a toddler, and Patsy from then on.

February 23 said, "You are Thelma, I am Louise. You are Lucy, I am Ethel. You are Elizabeth I, I am Mary, Queen of Scots—no, wait—"

And the last entry, on February 28, the day before I finished treatment, "Everything will be alright in the end. If it's not alright, it's not the end."

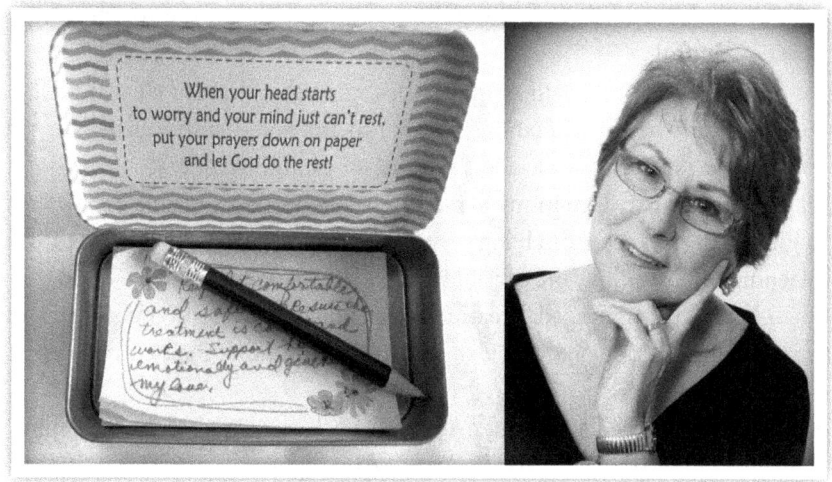

Prayer Box   Dorothy

During the second week post treatment I was disappointed that I wasn't getting better yet, but I told myself it was still early to expect significant improvement. I didn't leave the house because it was too painful if clothing touched my burns. It was March, cold, and I couldn't bear the weight of heavy outdoor clothing touching my skin. To perk myself up, I made one exception and rode along in the car with Chris when he delivered our yearly financial information to our tax accountant. That was the extent of my outside activity.

I was beginning to realize that during treatment it had been easier for me because I was actively engaged in fighting my disease and I was supported every day by people who helped with the fight. But when I was home alone the tendency to focus on negatives took over. I was so tired of the daily struggle by then, all the routines and efforts, and I wanted my normal life back. I tried not to show this to my family and friends, who wished me well and didn't deserve to be an object of my frustrations. But there were plenty of reasons to feel negative by then.

I was already applying creams to my skin every two hours to get through the day. Itching from my neck kept me awake most of the night. I got out of bed in the morning with my skin stuck to my pillow and blood on the pillowcase. I tried covering my pillow with a towel, but the rough texture was too painful.

Then I developed pain in my left ear again that drained clear fluid. Dr. Thomas said the inflammation was due to inner radiation burns like the exterior ones on my neck. He gave me an antibiotic that would prevent damage to the cartilage in my ear, and eardrops. After a couple of sleepless nights trying to keep from lying on my ear and trying to keep my neck from bleeding on my pillow, the ear got better.

I became discouraged. Treatment was finished. I was anxious to put all my struggles behind me and just get stronger. It didn't happen that way. I wasn't done yet.

Other side effects I'd gotten used to, such as skin dryness and splits, worsened. I was tired a lot from loss of sleep at night and general debilitation. Napping during the day made me feel even worse. I considered it a good day if I could spend an hour in my office and a couple of hours in front of the television at night.

I regained a tiny bit of my ability to taste food, but mucositis caused an overpowering salty taste and slimy feeling.

I was still getting worse instead of better. That realization came as a blow. And now I didn't have that daily crutch of talking to people who were experienced and cared for me. They had kept me going, but now I had to depend on myself.

Chris looked at me hopefully, standing by patiently but frustrated in his inability to make me feel better, watching for improvement that didn't come. I duly reported to family via the phone, trying to stay positive, minimizing some of what was really happening. Where was Robbie when I needed him? Where was Paul? Vani? Dr. Gold was on the East Coast. There was only me now.

March 11, 2018. My grandson, Aidan, played French horn with the Elgin Youth Symphony Orchestra. My first public outing since treatment began would be to attend Aidan's spring concert. We would attend the concert only and not make a long day by having a meal or socializing afterward. All I had to do was dress nicely, sit in the car for an hour while Chris drove us to Elgin, sit in a theater seat for another hour or so, and I could sleep on

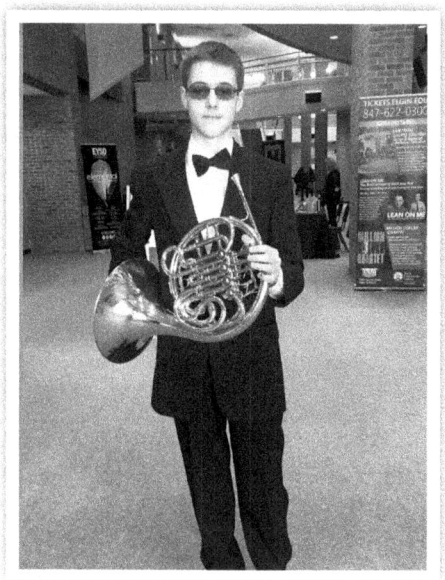

Aidan, Elgin Youth Symphony Orchestra, 2018

the ride home. Surely I could do that much. Hadn't I spent long days at the hospital, despite how bad I felt? Aidan was the only member of my family so far who seemed to have inherited my interest in performing music. I wanted to encourage that.

I remember only pieces of that day. I recall joining John and Clare in the vestibule of the performing venue while we all waited for the orchestra hall doors to open. There were a lot of people milling around. I had worn a comfortable dress and calf-length boots, so I was warm, and my neck didn't hurt too much. I thought I might have difficulty standing, but I didn't. After about twenty minutes the doors opened and we found our seats, right of center, two rows up on the second level, about thirty feet from the stage.

Several orchestras performed, first year students to advanced. The directors of each orchestra spoke about their group and then each group played a few pieces. I anxiously waited for Aidan's group, scheduled to perform last. When the students filed on stage, I raised my phone to film Aidan's arrival. I couldn't find him on the small screen and missed his entrance. In fact, at first I couldn't find him at all and had to ask Clare to point him out. There he was, my grandson, in the second row, and from that moment I watched and listened. What I heard was impressive. Proud grandma was too overwhelmed by the importance of the moment to do more than watch and listen. As a result, the only photo I took that day was one of Aidan, in a tuxedo and holding his horn, in the lobby of the theater after the program.

Then we returned home, with a sense of pride and accomplishment that rivaled confronting cancer. I didn't sleep on the ride home, but I did as soon as I got there.

Encouraged by my ability to attend Aidan's concert, I attempted to attend my first library board meeting the evening of March 13. That adventure didn't go quite as well. Although the meeting only took an hour, going out at night put me off schedule. I was unable to eat in the evening and spent the night dealing with nausea, but it was worth it. After almost three months away, seeing the other board members and contributing to the discussions that took place that evening was uplifting.

The third week post treatment was the low point of my entire treatment course. I faced the fact that I was still getting worse instead of better. Despite trying to talk myself into expecting an easy recovery, at that point I had had enough.

After all my efforts, after coming so far, I was at the point of giving up and going into a funk. What if, after months of agony, it had all been for nothing? What if I still had cancer?

The idea terrified me, and I pushed it out of my mind. I didn't want to get out of bed in the morning. I wanted to sleep to escape my fears. I wanted my life back! But there was nothing else I could do at that point. The treatment was over, the damage done. I had to stay confident in my ability to withstand the recovery period and struggle on.

My mouth was coated with mucus so thick and nasty in taste I was brought to near desperation. Every surface of my mouth was covered with slime. I had a powerful taste in my mouth that was salty, metallic, and cloyingly sweet all at the same time. It wouldn't go away. The mucus was thick and rubbery, hard to swallow and hard to spit out. I sometimes felt like I could put my hand in my mouth and pull it out.

I remembered that during my first visit to radiation oncology, Robbie and Dr. Gold had given me samples of MuGard, suggesting I take it right away to condition my mouth before the mucositis started. I did try MuGard then but wasn't convinced that it did anything because I didn't have mucositis at that time. Later, when the mucositis developed, I still didn't notice any change when I used it.

"Trust me," Robbie said. "If you hadn't been taking it, you would feel much worse than you do now."

Worse! I could barely imagine that. MuGard was syrupy in texture, and despite my altered taste buds it left a sickeningly sweet coating in my mouth that lasted for hours and made me queasy.

I reread the materials given to me on my last day of treatment and discovered to my horror that mucositis could last three months! As with other things, in the early days I had talked myself into believing that my mouth symptoms would be easily managed in the early days, when mucositis hadn't started yet, and then again later when it was mild. With so many concerns from the beginning, I hadn't sufficiently heeded Robbie's early warning that mucositis would last so long. Regrettably, I knew during recovery I had underrated how miserable I would become. For the first time I doubted my ability to keep trying. Then I remembered that Dr. Layan and Robbie had assured me that mucositis was self-limiting and would eventually resolve.

At this point I was spending two hours a day actively treating my radiation burns, and mouth care entailed brushing and using three mouth care products four times a day. My tongue, gums, and cheeks remained painful no matter what I did. I returned to oncology for an unscheduled visit to be sure I didn't have something else going on, but no, it was just mucositis. *Just!* I thought. Mucositis seemed to be the straw that would finally break me.

One night the salty taste was so overpowering I couldn't sleep, and the thought of having to deal with this for months longer seemed impossible. That was my emotional low point, the only time I thought I wanted to give up. But don't troubles always seem at their worst while tossing and turning during the night? In the morning, I found a new resolve and the next day, coincidentally, I was finally a little better, a turning point.

I wish I could sugar-coat (pun intended!) these mouth side effects, but I'd be lying if I did. I found them extremely difficult. The thought that mucositis could persist so long was depressing, but perhaps my refusal to believe the hard parts of cancer treatment from the beginning was a good thing for me, because not believing life would be so hard helped keep me from giving up. I preferred to think that normal was right around the corner.

Of course, my appetite had not yet returned, and I still couldn't enjoy food, but my sense of taste was slowly beginning to return. Sometimes I could recognize what was in my mouth, and I began testing little bits of food

I had considered "forbidden" up until then. Most didn't work out, but I kept testing, hoping one day for a better result.

My gums had turned white and the miserable, unpleasant taste was present night and day. I wondered if the symptoms seemed more acute because some of my taste was returning, whereas the intensity of the mucositis had been masked when I could barely taste at all. Nonetheless, I was sick of it all and just wanted my life back.

One thing I think helped me through these side effects, appetite, and eating difficulties was that I never lost the ability to smell, and I didn't avoid thinking about food. I read recipes and watched food commercials. I remembered favorite tastes and pictured myself enjoying particular foods. Although less satisfying, these measures gave me something to look forward to.

On March 19 I attended my first writers' group meeting. It may have been a bit too soon. I drove myself and was out for over two hours. I felt extremely weak when I got home. But having done something "normal" all on my own gave me a sense of accomplishment.

I was me again, at least for a little while.

It wasn't until week four post treatment that I was able to add back a few foods, very slowly, sampling a bite or two once or twice a day. I didn't get nauseous, but food still tasted bad. I got down little bites of meat, rice, vegetables, or bread if after chewing them I added water before swallowing, but I didn't enjoy eating because the mucus was still bad and the taste unpleasant. I kept experimenting. The burns on my neck were improving, and I was only lubricating my neck with Aquaphor ointment at night now.

Mucositis *wasn't* getting better yet, but thankfully it wasn't worsening. I took heart from the belief that it had peaked and would soon start to improve.

On March 21, three weeks after my cancer treatment finished, I had a video swallow evaluation. During that x-ray examination, Judith, my speech therapist, and a technician made films under fluoroscopy that showed how foods of varying consistencies traveled from my mouth to my stomach. When the test was completed, Judith gave me the results right away.

"You passed," she said with a smile. "We proved you're not aspirating.

You have no obstructions, no food is going into your airway, and your epiglottis is functioning normally. In other words, all your food is going to your stomach, not your lungs. However, due to radiation changes, some food isn't going *immediately* to your esophagus, but being held in what we term a 'safe' area."

"Is that dangerous?" I asked, my initial relief followed by alarm. Then I chuckled, realizing I had asked if "safe" was "dangerous."

"No. It only means you'll have to swallow more times to accomplish what one swallow used to do."

"Is that permanent? Will it get better? Or could it get worse?"

"Any of those things could happen. We just don't know. It depends on the exact areas of your radiation. Radiation affects everyone differently."

"What should I do?"

"Keep up the exercises you're already doing. You have to be careful when swallowing food, but you also have to swallow secretions all the time too. And remember that swallowing is the best exercise of all."

Judith must have noticed my concern. "Look, this is a good result. There's no indication you'll get worse, but stay on top of it as a precaution. You're good about that." She smiled.

I felt relieved that I had completed treatment without serious trouble swallowing. I had significant swelling in my neck, but the video swallow examination had shown that the muscles and structures in my throat were working properly. I had some discomfort, and some foods took more swallows, but it didn't appear likely that I would need a feeding tube in the future—unless late effects developed. As Judith advised, I continued to do swallowing exercises to be sure to protect that function, especially the hard swallows I found so difficult.

Although it took determination to keep up my blog every week without fail, it benefited me in many ways and turned out to be one of the best proactive decisions I made. My readers expected my posts to come every Tuesday. I didn't want to disappoint them. No matter how lousy I felt, I had to find time on a regular basis to think about and describe what was happening to me.

Although what I suffered was often negative, I don't think anyone would have been interested in, or benefited from, reading just about my complaints, whining, and angst, no matter how true that might be. I expected a good outcome and wanted to show that positivity. This desire forced me to think about my experience in a positive way, which was healthy. Writing the blog also gave me a sense of accomplishment, proving to myself I was able to do at least one worthwhile thing outside of taking care of my health. And I had the satisfaction of hoping that my words would help other cancer patients and the people who loved them.

I received comments and words of encouragement from people who read my blog, mentioning how brave I was. I never thought of myself as brave. I was just someone who wanted to live, who did whatever it took to increase those odds. I wanted a successful arrival at the end of my journey, but I also wished to make a difficult trip as easy as it could be. I hoped my words would help others understand what needed to be faced and be inspired to keep up their own efforts.

My endeavors, including the blog, seemed to be having the desired results. "You're doing well," I was told. "Keep doing the same thing. Keep in mind that if you weren't trying so hard, you'd feel even worse." It was reassuring, but slim comfort during the first month of recovery.

CHAPTER 41
Life Before Cancer: Mom Leaves Us, 2012

*I*t was Bob who talked to my mother about her final wishes. She was in the hospital again, with a bowel obstruction that time. Her surgeon would operate if she wished but cautioned against it due to her poor overall medical condition. Without the surgery she would die.

"Grandma," Bob said, holding her hand at her hospital bed, with me standing nearby, "the doctors need to know whether or not you want to have surgery."

"I don't want more surgery," she said. "I've had enough."

"Your bowel is not working. If your surgeon operates, you might get better. If he doesn't operate, you won't get better."

"Will I be in pain?"

"They'll be able to keep you comfortable. But you won't live."

She took a deep breath, then repeated, "I don't want more surgery. I've had enough."

"You can go into hospice then. But they can't keep you at the hospital if they aren't making you better, only comfortable. You don't need to be in the hospital for that."

I stepped to her side then. "Mom, you can come back home with us, and I'll get nurses to come in. Or you can go to a nursing home and nurses will be with you all the time. Chris and I will do whatever you want."

She looked at me. "I want to go home."

And so, we took her back to our house, got a hospital bed, and placed it in front of the television in the family room so we could be with her during the day. We hired round-the-clock nurses so someone knowledgeable could make her as comfortable as possible and suction her from the secretions she could no longer swallow that were making her struggle for breath.

Mom died in December 2012, at the age of ninety-three, ten days after she came back home.

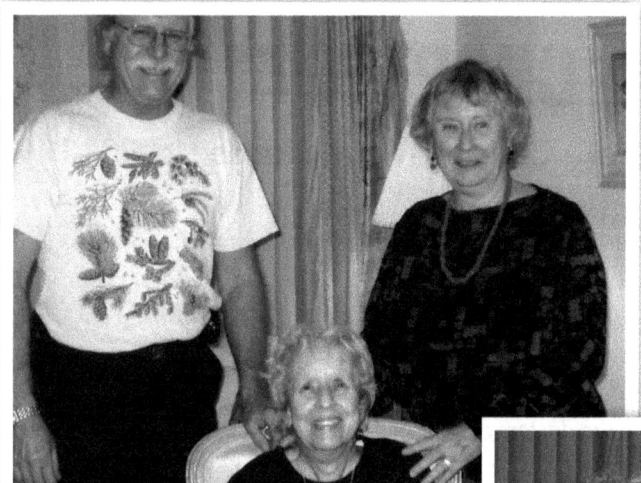

Mom's 90th Birthday:
Brother Mike, Mom, and me.

Mom's 90th Birthday, holding her wedding picture.

CHAPTER 42
Recovery, Month Two
April 2018

"You were done with radiation, but John said the radiation takes time to work its way out of the system, so you were still in a danger zone. I was disappointed to hear that, but the treatments at least were done." - Clare, daughter-in-law

"When you finished therapy, I was relieved that you wouldn't have to go through that anymore. To me it was a success." - John, son

"I was never concerned that you wouldn't make it. I was pretty sure you had the strength to do it." - Bob, son

I had the first sign of tongue cancer the previous Thanksgiving, was diagnosed shortly thereafter, started cancer treatment at the beginning of the year, finished it March 1, and by Easter I had finished one month of recovery. Four and a half months of "other life" and counting.

At my one-month follow-up visit after finishing therapy, my doctors thought I was doing well. I was happy with the way my burns were healing, but I was very disgusted with the mucositis and my inability to taste and enjoy food. My tongue hurt, especially at the tip. Mucositis stayed with me the longest of any of my side effects.

I only brushed and used Biotene for my mouth four times a day now, since my other mouth routines seemed to be doing more harm than good. Although I was still pretty miserable, these changes to my schedule gave me a little more personal time.

Despite the continued side effects, I gained strength and improved slowly. By Easter Sunday, April 1, which oddly happened to fall on April Fool's Day that year, I was able to enjoy Easter Day brunch with my family. Everyone pitched in to do the work. I rather liked this point-and-watch-others-work approach to holiday meals. I'd have to think about how to arrange that for future holidays!

I nibbled a little food, taking a bite or two of ham and French toast casserole. Sadly, the blueberry shortcake with fresh whipped cream I had looked forward to tasted excessively sour to my altered taste buds. Nonetheless, I sat at the table with a plate in front of me and my family around me, and it seemed like a normal holiday.

Although we color eggs for Easter like many families, the tradition in our family is to hunt for Easter baskets. We would prepare a number of baskets—anywhere from four to seven—and hide them throughout the house.

This was the first time Mia was old enough to enjoy the hunt. With Daddy Bob close behind coaching and snapping pictures on his phone, Mia—so cute in a little black-and-white-pinstriped dress and little white patent-leather shoes—squealed every time she found a basket. Baskets were filled with plastic eggs with little treats inside, a limited amount of candy, and toys and books from the dollar store. Mia was following in Grandma's footsteps, already an avid reader like I had been at her age.

Then we stood Mia next to Big Bunny, a four-foot-tall, pudgy pink blow-up bunny that we'd inflated every year since John and Bob were toddlers. The whole family took pictures with our phones, intending this to be the first of many Easter-with-Big-Bunny pictures over the years.

With caution, my energy level lasted through mid-afternoon, when everyone left for their homes. Chris and I settled down in front of the television and nodded off. It had been a tiring day for me, even if only half a day. I was disappointed that I couldn't taste the food we'd made but encouraged by the fact that I had at least had a few bites without getting sick.

Easter was the first day I went entirely off the pain medications I'd been taking to that point. I had taken the minimum I needed to be able to sleep and eat up until then, but I still considered it a milestone to be able to stop them entirely. I did feel a little worse than normal that night, but I didn't return to pain pills again.

The Wednesday after Easter, April 4, I saw my doctors for the first time since I finished treatment.

I greeted Dr. Layan with a wry comment. "Now I know why you scheduled my first post-treatment visit a whole month after I finished radiation therapy. You didn't want to hear me cussing you out and wanted to wait until I'd plateaued or turned the corner." We laughed together.

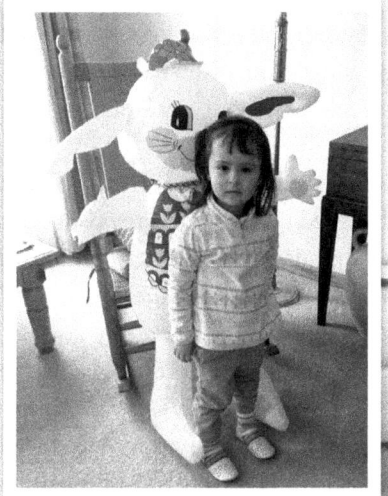

Mia, Easter 2018

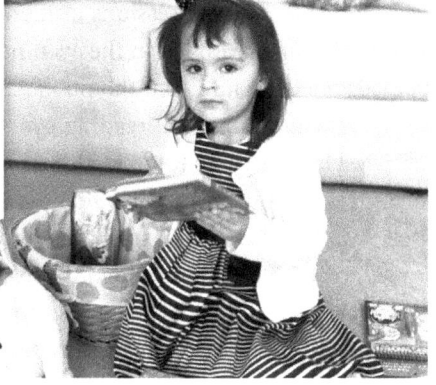

After Easter I slowly began a major turning point. Soon I was encouraged by enough improvement in my energy level to think about resuming full normal activities, and I slowly began to pick them up again. I began to think about things other than cancer.

Again I realized it had been a good thing that I underestimated the first month of recovery. I may have been depressed if I hadn't fooled myself into thinking that recovery would be immediately uphill. Recovery was a big deal, bigger even than treatment, but my error gave me something to look forward to. Then, by the time I started to realize the worst was over at last, normal life seemed doable again and I was uplifted from my funk.

By early April, almost six weeks post treatment, my neck burns were still uncomfortable, but I could wear soft clothing and get out in public again. My skin was what I would describe as "normally dry," and the "snakeskin" and "splits" were gone. My throat was still very dry and hurt when I swallowed, especially in the afternoon and evening. Mucositis was as bad as ever. My sense of taste returned a little, but I still had no appetite. Everything still tasted metallic and salty, but I was able to eat small portions of whatever I cooked for Chris. I ate mostly oatmeal, but now I was eating grits as well. Not enjoying grits much, but at least it was a change from old reliable oatmeal. I was glad I wasn't like a patient Dr. Layan told me about who was only able to eat watermelon.

By the beginning of April, my weight had dropped by thirty pounds. That was a compromise between where I wished I was and where my doctors wanted me to be. I returned to working Wednesdays at the Lemont Historical Society archives, short sessions at first. I got tired by midafternoon, but I tried to stay awake longer in the evenings.

I decided I could face the public again and agreed to do a reading at my writers' group annual reading event on April 8 at the Downers Grove Library. I knew that after talking for a short time, my dry mouth could either turn speech to a rasp, my voice would give out entirely, or I'd have a coughing spell. I was nervous about speaking in front of an audience, but a friend had agreed to complete my reading if I couldn't do so.

I selected two short passages from my novel, *The Mystery at Black Partridge Woods*, one reading from present day and one in the voice of my main historical character, a Potawatomi woman. I would need to talk non-stop for five or six minutes. Could I do that? Tired of living my life around my health, I was determined to try.

When I arrived at the library, I was greeted by a friend, a fellow writer I hadn't seen since my cancer diagnosis. "You look great," he said. "No one would ever know you had cancer. You must be glad it's all over."

I bit my tongue, smiled, and thanked him. He was a nice guy who was trying to give me a compliment. But inside I seethed. *It's not over! Not by a long shot! I look "great" because I lost thirty pounds, and I made a supreme effort to dress well and wear make-up. Inside I'm more miserable than I could ever tell you. No way was what I went through anywhere near as easy as you think.*

Throughout my struggle I had found myself trying not to get annoyed by friends who called with positive attitudes. Their "helpful" suggestions just didn't fit what was happening to me. Didn't they realize how sick I felt? How sick I still was? Didn't they know my cancer could return? That I could die? That, after all I'd been through, I would still fear those possibilities?

I soon calmed down. After all, I hadn't realized myself how really hard cancer was going to be. How could I expect others to?

When it was my turn at the podium, I spoke slowly and carefully, taking sips of water as needed. I didn't lose my voice, and I didn't cough, although my voice was weak and my throat felt strained by the time I finished.

It was what happened after the readings, when I approached the snack table, that the really big moment occurred. As I sampled a bite here and a bite there, expecting no joy from the experience, I picked up a slice of green pepper and scooped some dip with it. Up to this point, I had avoided raw vegetables, which were especially unappetizing, but I was determined to keep trying a variety of foods.

I couldn't believe it! A faint taste of what I remembered as green pepper washed over my tongue! The dip was completely lost, but the pepper! Something I could recognize—something real! Tears sprang to my eyes. A friend came up and touched my arm. "Is everything okay?" he said.

"More than okay," I said. "This is so good!"

He eyed me strangely. I was swooning, tears in my eyes, over green pepper? "O…kay," he said, made his excuses, and escaped, perhaps suspecting that cancer had addled my brain.

Would I taste cucumber too? I tried. No, not cucumber. No joy there. Celery? A little better, but not like the pepper. Carrot? Not yet. I put pepper after pepper on my plate, leaving little for anyone else, but I didn't care. I had never enjoyed the fresh crunch, the moist flow across my tongue, as I enjoyed that pepper. I could hardly wait to get home and share the moment with Chris. And send him to the store for green peppers.

After that, I continued to gradually increase my activities. I began walking the indoor track again to build strength.

I still ate oatmeal for the most part, but I stopped drinking Ensure. I couldn't eat acidic, strong-flavored, or overly sweet foods at all—foods like salad dressings, ketchup, or chocolate. I could eat small portions of meat, bread, rice, potatoes, nuts, vegetables, and other bland foods. My appetite had not returned yet, and the mucositis coating, tongue irritation, and taste function were as bad as ever. Eating was still an unpleasant chore instead of enjoyable. My ability to swallow normally got a bit stronger, and I could even repeat-swallow—if I did it carefully, so I didn't start a coughing spell.

Usually, I woke up about eight in the morning. It took an hour or so to regain my voice and get moving. Then I could count on four or five pretty good hours of activity, if I paced myself. By midafternoon I'd start to tire, and my voice would give out along with my energy level.

But hey! I had a half day now, and I could shift my routines such that they gave me some usable time. Yeah, so I still didn't feel so great. I was functioning. It was a beginning.

A problem with returning to public activities is that there's a difference between how you view what you can or can't do and how the people you work with view you. You want to prove to yourself that you're able to function, but it's a real effort to make yourself look good and perform in your former capacity. Your effort creates the impression on others that you feel good and can do everything you did before at the same level. People sometimes push you to do things you can't do yet and don't understand that it's not that you won't, but that you *can't*. Because you've made that effort to look good, some people don't believe your explanations and think you're making excuses.

For instance, volunteers at the historical society might suggest ideas that required my involvement. They might be very good suggestions.

"That's a great idea," I'd say. "But unfortunately, I'm going to have to put that on the backburner. I'm just not up to it yet."

I could tell from the looks on their faces that they thought I was making an excuse.

Since I no longer had daily medical appointments and was home all day, before I got too involved with activities outside the home, I spent some time trying to straighten out papers that had piled up in my office. I worked little by little, a half hour or so at a time, and quit when I felt myself getting tired.

A few weeks after I started treatment, I began receiving explanations of benefits, or EOBs, from my insurers, Medicare and BlueCross BlueShield. I had set them aside to look at later, when I felt well enough to face them. I hadn't realized at first that we hadn't gotten any bills, since I knew my health care providers would bill my insurance first and it would be months before any remaining charges would arrive in the mail.

Understanding how payers and patients shared the high costs of medical care had been a major part of my job when I worked at Rush. For that reason, when the EOBs finally arrived, I studied them. It was easier for me than for most patients to decipher what they meant.

When we retired and started receiving Medicare benefits, Chris and I had purchased the best secondary plan available from BlueCross BlueShield of Illinois. We wanted nothing to do with alternate options that involved oversight by HMO or PPO plans. I had helped too many patients throughout the years who couldn't see the doctors they wanted to see or go to the hospitals that offered the treatment they preferred or who were denied options that their doctors thought best for them by their insurers. Often these people got stuck with huge bills, or their outcome was poor because they were denied some part of their care for a cheaper, but less effective, alternative. Sometimes they went to a hospital or doctor who wasn't in their plan. Whether they did that knowingly or unknowingly, it made no difference—they still had reduced coverage and paid more themselves.

We paid a lot of money for our insurance. Fortunately, we were in a position to do so. Freedom of choice, when it came to health, was not a luxury but a necessity in my mind. So we scrimped on other things and paid for the best insurance.

When I looked over the EOBs at last, despite my experience, I was stunned by the high costs of my treatment. I was relieved to discover that every penny allowed was being paid by Medicare and BlueCross BlueShield, leaving me with no financial responsibility. I was also astonished by the amount I would have had to pay from our savings if we hadn't purchased the best insurance available. I felt sorry for people who didn't have good coverage. If I had to worry about paying many thousands of dollars on top of the misery of my cancer treatment, if I wasn't able to choose Rush and the research study option, I can't imagine how much harder my life would have been with those additional worries.

I was thankful I didn't have to limit my choices and could let my doctors decide what was best for me.

April 12 was a beautiful day, the sort of day we looked forward to at this time of year—rare, but this is Chicago, with its weather mixture of dreary, miserable, and lovely. The book I had set aside when I got cancer,

The Mystery at Mount Forest Island, was set in a remote off-trail location in the Palos Forest Preserves, a place that was once a golf course operated in the 1920s to 1940s by the Cook County Forest Preserves. The abandoned course had the added mystique of having been a place where Al Capone, an avid golfer, had once played, and later became the site of the Manhattan Project when the world's first nuclear reactor was moved to those woods from the University of Chicago.

I had been to the location before with a brother and sister who had grown up in a farmhouse where the course's caretaker had lived. When we visited the former site of those buildings, nothing remained but wilderness, with little sign that anything else had ever been there.

Another friend of mine did a lot of off-trail exploring. He found remnants of the buildings and invited me to visit them with him. I wanted to see what he found. Time was crucial, since once the foliage leafed out, anything that remained would be much harder to find. For me this was another first: the first time I tried to walk on an extended hike, part of it uphill. I liked walking uphill about as much as I liked exercise—not at all. But, if I wanted to start writing that book again—*finishing* that book—I had to take the opportunity, and I didn't want to wait until November when the shrubs were bare again.

So Chris and I met Ken in the parking lot at Saganashkee Slough. Ken was a tall, attractive man in his forties, a quiet and rather shy man who had an avid interest in exploring the backcountry and history of the area between Willow Springs and Lemont. I followed a Facebook page he wrote and thought he probably knew more than anyone else about the area, since he spent so much time tracking down details, doing research, and then exploring the trails and wilderness, relating what he found to the past.

Ken eased out of his pickup truck, wearing camouflage pants and hiking boots, carrying a walking stick he had fashioned from a twisted tree branch. We smiled, happy to be together sharing a common passion. After a few moments of small talk, Chris and I followed Ken across 107th Street to an old, chained-off service road that climbed the bluff of what historians called Mount Forest Island. The entire triangular-shaped area extended about five miles at its widest points, and had once been an island in ancient Lake Chicago, the body of glacial waters that later drained to become Lake Michigan. Now the former island was almost completely filled by the Palos Forest Preserves, and the shore of Lake Michigan was some thirty miles to the east.

The area looked different this time without the summer foliage that hid the remains of the demolished golf clubhouse and farm we had come to find. I used a trekking pole to help me with the hill, and the men paced themselves so I could keep up with them. Ken pointed out the depression and concrete blocks that remained where the basement of the farmhouse had been and then the foundation of an adjacent pole barn. A huge poplar tree still marked the spot that we had missed when I visited the year before with the former residents of the farm.

Then we walked to where the clubhouse had stood, about a quarter mile away. We saw flagstones lining the service road, which had once led to the golf course. In spots, pavers were exposed that had been salvaged from Roosevelt Road and reused for the entrance road. We found part of the concrete foundation of the demolished clubhouse and a few pieces of red clay tiles from the clubhouse roof. I took pictures of everything. I could go there and find these things myself now. I could use my experience to inspire my book. Excited by the project, I knew I would soon be writing, my work no longer set aside but a part of my life again.

During April I sent out three blogs: One about nutrition and speech therapy, one about my medical providers, and one about my early recovery period.

So how did I feel as the end of April approached?

Well, I wished I felt better.

I wished that the next day I would feel like I felt before I got cancer.

I really wanted a Big Mac, a piece of pizza, and a glass of wine that I could taste.

I wished I didn't feel so tired late in the day and that it wasn't so hard to go to meetings in the evening.

I wished I didn't have to struggle to talk between sips of water and a painful, dry mouth.

I wished I could spend a full day on normal activities.

I wished my throat didn't hurt and I could enjoy eating again.

I wished I didn't cough so much.

On the positive side:

I was happy to be well enough to start returning to activities I enjoyed: family, writing, volunteer and board activities.

Pain and nausea, although they remained to some degree, no longer interfered substantially with my life.

I could eat and swallow, but not yet enjoy, some food, and my skin was almost normal again.

I didn't "crash" physically as early in the day or as often.

I was starting to consider scheduling social events and personal appearances again.

My calendar was starting to list more than medical appointments. It had things I was looking forward to.

I had a new wardrobe, composed substantially of old clothes that now fit me.

I felt that I accomplished something big and worthwhile, and that I met a challenge with a positive attitude and grace.

I felt it was possible to finish the book I had started.

I was optimistic again.

I was considering joining my chorus on their planned trip to New York to perform at Carnegie Hall in June.

A new determination hit me. *Whatever it takes, I'm going to enjoy a Big Mac. Or a plate of lasagna, maybe with a glass of wine. Or Chris and I will go out to a restaurant. I will publish more historical mysteries about my hometown, and maybe I will write a book about my journey through head and neck cancer. I will not let these opportunities pass! And I will sing at Carnegie Hall!*

"The long black skirt is classic, but the navy mid-calf with the paisley border print is dated," Clare, my daughter-in-law, said, then looked at me apologetically. "Don't be angry with me…" She was afraid I'd think she was being ruthless.

By the end of April, I was still losing weight. With the thirty pounds and counting I lost since cancer entered my life, my clothes didn't fit anymore. For years I had boxed up favorite clothes that had gotten too tight, thinking someday I might fit them again. Well, "someday" was here! If they were ever going to be of any use, now was the time to wear them or get rid of them once and for all.

I pulled boxes out of storage and tried the old clothes on. They fit, but were they fashionable enough? Were they suitable for a woman my age? I was many years younger when I packed them away.

Had this gray linen suit I loved come back in style? Was it classic enough to wear again? Maybe I could alter it. Was the color and fabric out of fashion? Would Goodwill even want it? All my pants had wide legs and skinny pants were the style. Can a woman my age wear skinny pants or leggings? I didn't trust my ability to put outfits together. What shoes did I wear with the current styles? I had no dress boots at all, only snow boots.

I wasn't good at this, but Clare had a masters in fashion design, so I asked her for help.

"We'll figure this out," Clare said. She noticed the gray linen suit I'd been looking at and picked it up. "Here. Why don't you slip this on, and we'll see how it looks?"

After I put on the suit, Clare put her hands on my shoulders and stood me in front of a full-length mirror. "What do you think?"

My eyes filled with tears. Despite lack of makeup, the wrong shoes for the suit, and my current bad hairstyle, I looked good!

Two hours later, exhausted from taking clothes on and off, I was pleased. I had more useful clothes than I'd thought. Nonetheless, Goodwill was going to have to open an annex.

Ask any woman—one of life's greatest satisfactions is putting on a terrific outfit, looking in the mirror, and thinking you look good.

CHAPTER 43
Remission
May 2018

"When your treatment was over, it was still wait and see. We wanted to be sure it worked, and that takes additional testing with scans and physical examinations by ENT." - Bob, son

"It's normal for people who are losing weight and uncomfortable because they are ill to be crabby and grumpy, but I didn't see that in you. You expressed the unpleasantness, but you didn't snap at people or cry." - Clare, daughter-in-law

"I bought you new clothes because you needed something to cheer you up and take your mind off it." - Dolly, daughter-in-law

"Dr. Thomas said you looked pretty good, some swelling that seemed to be going down. I was pretty confident that they had gotten hold of it."
- Chris, husband

By the beginning of May, my third month of recovery, I was pretty discouraged. I felt stronger, but I still had mucositis, dry mouth, poor taste, skin sensitivity and swelling—especially around my throat—and days when I just didn't feel well. I tired easily, productive only half of each day. I was sick from the disease, but also sick of thinking about fighting cancer every day. I was tired of dreading eating instead of enjoying eating.

STAYING ALIVE IS A LOT OF WORK: ME AND MY CANCER

I wanted my life back.

I wanted a glass of wine!

My biggest fear was that, after all this, my cancer might not be gone. Did I go through months of sickness and pain only to find out I still had cancer and needed further treatment? A PET scan would tell me that, but I couldn't get it until three months after my treatment ended. If I got it sooner than that, before sufficient healing had taken place, I could have had false positive results. No one wanted to have further treatment based on false positive results. I had to wait.

"Oh, I'm so sorry!" well-intentioned friends and relatives said at the beginning of my cancer. "But you're strong. I hope you'll feel well soon."

That's not the way cancer works. With cancer, you often start off feeling well and treatment makes you sick. To get rid of your disease, you have to suffer side effects that aren't nice and aren't easy. You don't get better every day, you get worse every day, and that continues months after treatment is over. It's a slow and depressing process.

One day in early May, Chris found me sitting in an easy chair in our guest room, Mom's old room, the same chair I escaped to when I felt sick in the night. I was staring out the window at the Bradford pear tree in our front lawn, which had finished blooming for the season.

"Are you okay?" Chris asked, standing in the doorway.

"Yeah," I said. "Just thinking."

"About?"

"About surprises."

He came into the room and sat at the end of the guest bed, facing me.

"And?"

"Everything has been a surprise since I got this thing."

"The cancer thing?"

"Yeah. It surprised me that I got it. Remember how I wouldn't believe it?"

"I think that's normal, right?"

"I suppose. I was surprised at how it took over my whole life and so many parts of my body, not just my tongue and mouth. Surprised when I actually got the side effects everybody *told me* I'd get, and surprised about how they went on and on. And, on the other hand, surprised that I didn't vomit or have as much pain as I expected. I worked in the medical field all my life. You'd think I'd know what would happen. But I didn't."

"Is that a problem?"

"Not really. Were you surprised too?"

He shrugged and looked out the window. "I was surprised when Dr. Earvolino felt your neck and said she didn't like what she felt. Otherwise, I didn't know what to expect. We just did what we had to do."

I reached over and squeezed his knee.

As May started, the weather warmed and buds bloomed outside my windows, hinting at better times ahead. Say what one might about the challenges of Chicago's weather, as each new season began there were aspects of the season that I looked forward to. I saw winter as a time to appreciate the warmth and peacefulness of my home, a time to declutter and accomplish personal tasks that had piled up, a time to cuddle under a blanket, read, or snooze, and I looked forward to those things. Then as the long winter droned on, I tired of being indoors, facing wind, snow, ice, and brutal temperatures, bundled in layers of thick, heavy clothes. As spring began, I longed to toss off the heavy clothing, expose my face and my skin to the sun and warm breezes, get out and walk in my garden, in my neighborhood, or in the nearby forest preserves, see my friends and neighbors outside their homes again.

That spring the longing was more poignant than in previous years. The realization that I had survived a frightening time, a dangerous time, even life itself, was inspiring. I appreciated my life in a new way and was grateful for the little things that appear in spring, such as the unknown sprouts pushing through the flowerbeds, the bulbs squirrels had planted as surprises in unexpected places. My love for trees had prompted me to plant too many around our home, but they were in their full glory as I walked in the sun and said hello to my dogwoods, crabapples, redbuds, maples, and tree peonies.

"I'm back!" I told each plant. I believed life would be better for me, and that "my time" was almost here at last.

My PET scan on May 16 didn't show any remaining—or new—cancer. My doctors were all smiles when they gave me the news. I smiled too, happy of course, and relieved. But I didn't cry with happy tears, nor did I feel any really strong emotion. Much as I wanted to end cancer treatment on a joyful note—"Yay, world! I'm cured!"—it would not have been how I really felt.

Almost since my cancer treatment began, I'd been dreaming of the day and forming sentences in my mind for how I would tell the world I was in remission, or cancer-free. I imagined calling all my family and friends, sending out the good news on my blog, finding a happy picture and putting it on Facebook. When the time came, and the good news, I felt numb and didn't know how to react. I only told close family. Me, the writer—I had no words. I didn't know what to say, how to say it, who to say it to. So I said nothing at first. I can't explain why I reacted that way. After all, this was the most important thing to happen since my diagnosis. The PET scan was positive confirmation that my treatment had worked and there was no sign of cancer anywhere in my body. Up until the scan was read, we hadn't known if all our efforts had been worthwhile.

Maybe I didn't celebrate because, just as I was unwilling to admit at the beginning that I *had* cancer, I was then unwilling to admit I *no longer* had cancer. Perhaps I felt it was premature to say I was cancer-free, because being in remission meant although I no longer had any signs or symptoms of cancer, no evidence of disease on examination or my PET scan, undetectable cancer cells could remain in my body.

Maybe I didn't want to say the words in case what I said turned out to be wrong. Maybe, once again, I didn't believe what I was being told. Or others might not think my news was important and I would be disappointed by their reaction. It seemed too private a matter and, truth be told, a bit scary.

Or maybe I didn't like change, didn't like to say goodbye to cancer like I hated to say goodbye to family, friends, or other things that had become part of my life and I'd had to leave behind.

Cancer was a momentous event in my life, and it was over. I hoped. Telling people makes it real. Perhaps I didn't feel confident enough to make that statement.

Or maybe it was because, although I was grateful and functional, I couldn't yet get my head around how having cancer had changed my life. Or maybe I resisted change, even in the right direction.

My life slowly returned to some semblance of normality, but a new normality with physical, emotional, and medical restrictions. My life wasn't exactly as it had been, but I had a reasonable quality of life. I looked forward to the future, but it was becoming clear that some of the effects of my cancer and its treatment might always be with me, and some new problems could even crop up in years to come—late effects, they're called.

I'm as guilty as the next guy in thinking, when I meet someone who tells me their cancer is in remission, "I'm so sorry you had cancer, but you're well and it's over, right?" No, that comment is *not* right. Those fortunate enough to be in remission will have periodic check-ups, suffer continued—and even new—side effects, have burdensome daily health routines, and perhaps medications that may have their own side effects. They will *always* worry about the cancer coming back. After five years free of cancer, their doctor will usually pronounce them "cured," but that only lets them back off a bit, since the threat of cancer will always be there, maybe not the same cancer but a new one.

True, the threat of cancer is there for people who have not had cancer too. The difference is that if you haven't had cancer, you don't really know what it is you're dreading. I was monitored, at first monthly, then with decreasing frequency. Every time I waited anxiously for the results of my examinations or tests. NED—no evidence of disease—that's what I wanted to hear. And that was what I continued to hear.

Physically and mentally, I progressed well. A few days before my PET scan we had gone on the first short vacation I'd been able to take, driving to Fort Wayne to spend a long weekend with Bob, Dolly, and Mia for Mother's Day. It was good to do something that had nothing to do with cancer, and all went well on the trip.

During our stay in Fort Wayne, Dolly had taken me to a mall to visit my favorite clothing stores and spent way too much on me.

"You have enough big and baggy clothes," she said. "You need some things that fit."

Four months after I finished therapy, I tried to stay positive, but sometimes I still got discouraged. Throughout my life, when I got sick, I'd eventually heal and life would return to normal, the sickness a thing of the past and forgotten. But I wasn't ready yet to accept that some of my side effects would be permanent.

I wished I could just flip a switch and life would be like it was before.

I wished I could enjoy eating again. I could eat most foods by May, but eating wasn't yet a pleasurable experience. I was gradually tasting more. Every single time I thought about eating I expected the taste to be what I remembered. Then I put the food in my mouth, and now and then the taste was similar, but usually that initial taste was unreliable and lasted for only a few bites, and then the customary bitter, rancid taste would fill my mouth, disappointing me again. *Every time.* Some foods I still couldn't eat, such as spicy or acidic foods like pizza or pineapple. It took much longer for me to eat, and I needed about a pint of water with each meal to be able to swallow my food due to dryness from impaired salivary glands. I still ate oatmeal almost every morning.

In an earlier chapter I mentioned that I was looking forward to a Big Mac and a glass of wine. I could take some sips of wine, but not a whole glass yet. I could eat hamburgers with limited condiments if they weren't too thick. The muscles in my jaw sustained some radiation impairment that limited how far I could open my mouth to bite something thick like a hamburger, but chewing was fine.

I'd made a lot of progress. I was eating a reasonable quantity of food and stopped losing weight. I could swallow pretty well, but sometimes liquids trickled down my throat and started me coughing. My throat was still irritated, but less painful, and my mouth was no longer sensitive. The mucositis was pretty much a thing of the past. Thank God for that! My tongue was still a bit discolored and felt fuzzy, a probable consequence of dry mouth. The dryness was likely to be with me for life.

I was once again getting out into the world socially. I attended another of Aidan's concerts in Elgin on May 6 and Collin's high school graduation on May 27, and those times I was able to stay for a dinner celebration afterward, although I had to be careful what I ate. My energy level was building, and I was staying up most of the day by then.

I had resumed library board and committee obligations and regular Wednesday morning volunteer hours at the historical society. I tired more easily, but I finished what I wanted to do, came home, rested, and started the next day without difficulty, if not exactly *fresh*.

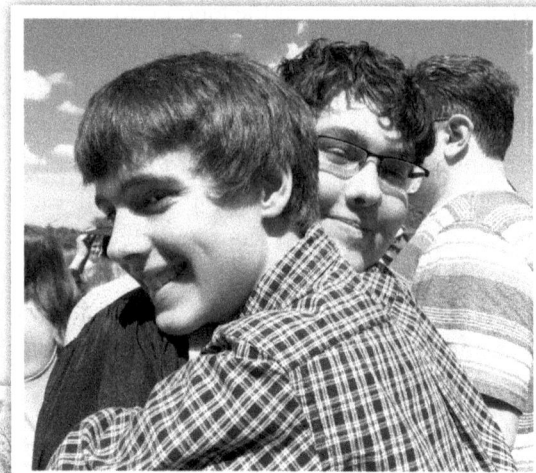

Collin and Aidan

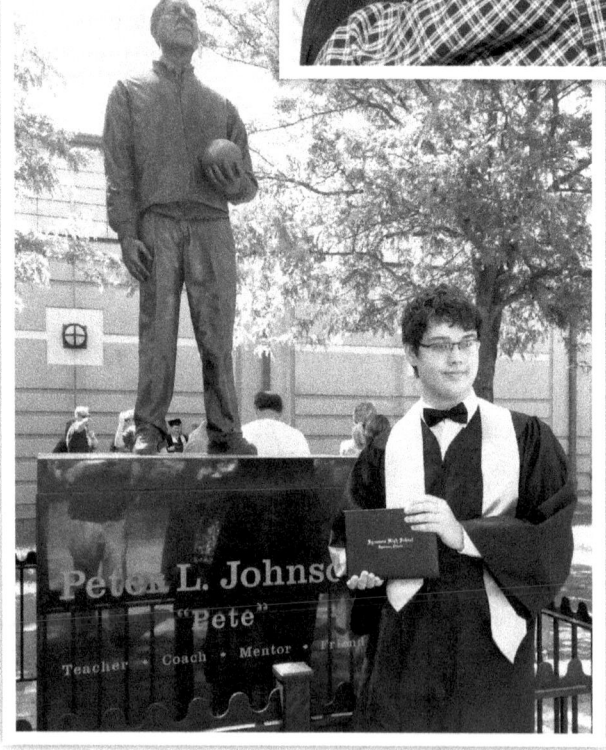

Collin, High School Graduation, 2018

CHAPTER 44
Life Before Cancer:
Chris and I, Alone Again, 2013-2017

*A*fter Mom died, Chris and I were alone again. We missed Mom, but it was a relief to finally have our lives to ourselves. We were looking forward to a bright future.

I gathered the materials I had set aside during Mom's final illness and threw all my energies into completing my first marketable work, a historical mystery novel titled The Mystery at Sag Bridge. My intent was, if no one liked it I would give up my aspirations of a writing career, with no tears shed since I was already involved in other satisfying activities.

I finished my first novel in mid-2014 and started looking for a publisher. I took a one-week course to learn how to develop a "query," studied the market, and sent off my first batch—ten queries to agents, and ten queries to publishers. I didn't receive a single response from agents, but four publishers were interested in my book. I rejected two: one because I didn't think they were right for my book and another because their process was too long. Between the final two, I selected Amika Press because they were in Chicago, had a personal touch, and promised to have my book in print within six months. I never regretted that decision.

It turned out people liked my books. The Mystery at Sag Bridge *came out* in April of 2015. I got good reviews and fan letters.

The Mystery at Sag Bridge *and my new career as a writer weren't the best things born in 2015. Three months after my book was published, Dolly gave birth to my only granddaughter, Mia. I wished I had more time to spend with her. They lived three hours away, but we visited as often as we could.*

The Mystery at Sag Bridge *did pretty well. I started being invited to local events, to book clubs, and to speak at libraries and in the community. Then, in August 2016, I published* The Mystery at Black Partridge Woods.

Everyone had warned me that promoting books was a lot more time-consuming than I could imagine, and they were right. At first, I was reluctant to speak to an audience, but I created some lectures about the historical periods in my books and sought out libraries and historical societies to speak to. I found that I enjoyed meeting people and sharing my work and my knowledge of local history with them. And so, with two novels under my belt, book discussion groups, author events, and public speaking were taking up any free time I might have.

I was a senior citizen. All my adult life I'd had obligations. I'd had a fulfilling and rewarding career. I'd raised two successful sons I was proud of. I had two wonderful daughters-in-law and three gifted grandchildren. I had a supportive husband I loved. I'd been through trial by fire providing care and support to my elderly parents.

I was free at last!

Free from those burdens, I started to believe that "my time" had finally come. The time Chris and I could devote, not to responsibilities for others, but to our own passions. I had made a promising start by involving myself in activities I'd always longed to do. I'd successfully published two historical mystery novels.

My new activities kept me busy, perhaps too much so. In fact, I was busier writing and promoting than I had ever been as a medical group administrator at Rush, and I had thought that was impossible. But surely, I could learn how to say no at last.

And, thankfully, I had never been seriously ill myself.

CHAPTER 45
Carnegie Hall
June 2018

"When I watched you on stage at Carnegie Hall, I was pleased to see you in your comfort zone, doing something you loved. I remember thinking things were going to be okay." – Bob, son

I would probably never have an opportunity to sing in Carnegie Hall again.

Whether I was strong enough to make the trip and if my dry mouth and hoarseness would allow me to sing was questionable. I had finished radiation and chemotherapy only three months before. My burns were healed, but I still had swelling around my voice box, tired easily, and my appetite remained poor. Eating in restaurants would be a problem too.

But I had to try.

It had been a long time since Chris and I traveled by plane. The unfamiliarity with booking planes online almost defeated me. Bob, who traveled often, took pity on me. We made reservations at the host hotel, and Bob sent me step-by-step instructions for booking air travel. He would be arriving by car a few hours before the concert with Dolly and Mia, now three years old. They would stay for a few days after the concert, and we would enjoy New York City as a family.

Chris and I arrived at our hotel in New York on May 30. The company that produced the concert was organized and the director talented. All I had to do was know the music, show up, and follow directions.

The first rehearsal in the hotel ballroom took place the afternoon following our arrival.

"I guess I'll wander around and explore while you're practicing," Chris said.

"It's not practice, it's rehearsal," I said.

He shot me one of those looks that clearly meant it was the same thing and quit being a know-it-all.

"Practice is something I do alone, to learn the music. We're expected to know it already. Rehearsal is when we all come together to perform as a group. It's different."

He rolled his eyes, clearly not seeing a difference. "Whatever. If I'm not here when you get back, call me on my cell. I'll be nearby."

I attended two three-hour rehearsals in a convention hall in our hotel, the first the afternoon of June 1 and the second the following morning. A couple of times during rehearsals, I felt a screech instead of a note about to emerge. When that happened, I just moved my mouth along with the other singers.

"I'm doing this," I said under my breath. "I'm going to sing in Carnegie Hall!" I hoped the director wouldn't notice me and feared he would ask me to withdraw. It's hard to hide, even in a large chorus, from a director. They hear everything!

Part of my enjoyment in singing classical music came from learning the history of the work. The Austrian composer, Joseph Haydn, perhaps the most prolific composer of all time, was commissioned to write the Mass we were singing for the 600th anniversary of the famous pilgrimage church, Mariazell. It was his third rendition of the piece, which was first written in 1766, lost in a fire, and recreated from his memory in 1768. Ironically, this third, enduring version was not performed at Mariazell due to a lack of suitable musicians, but instead in Vienna in 1782. That version of the Mass survived to be enjoyed to this day.

From the first moment of rehearsal, I was captured by the loveliness of the music, the skill of the director—who was new to me—and the voices of the soloists. The orchestra would not join us until our dress rehearsal.

On the morning of the performance, Chris and I walked to Carnegie Hall from our nearby hotel to be sure there would be no last-minute glitches at dress rehearsal. We found the backstage entrance and then walked to the front to check out the box office and the billboard.

I stepped to the sign and lifted my arm, pointing at our group, the Downers Grove Choral Society. At that moment, seeing my chorus's name in letters at the hall, reality hit me. This was no longer a dream. I was actually here. I burst into a grin and turned to Chris as he took a picture with my phone.

Later that afternoon, I arrived at the backstage entrance for dress rehearsal, pass in hand, imprinted with the date, time, and my name. I showed the pass at the door. Chris gave me a kiss and walked away.

Our dressing room, we had been told, was on the second floor. I walked through what looked to me like any large time-worn office building, past a staircase into an area with a few elevators. I joined others in the elevator, got off, and wandered down the hall, looking for any face I knew. The long, crowded hallway passed many doors and branches. The clean, off-white walls, unlike those found in other old hallways, were hung with posters of previous headliners: Tchaikovsky, Dvorak, Mahler, Gershwin, Maria Callas, Judy Garland, The Beatles. Now, Pat Camalliere was here, awed to be in the same place as these notable music giants.

I finally spotted a few members of our chorus gathered farther down the hall and headed in that direction, my steps ticking over red-oak-colored hard industrial flooring.

Inside, our dressing room was a continuation of clean white walls and posters of famous musicians. There were racks for our belongings and there was a piano, but few chairs for the hundred people in the room.

We lined up in the order that had been determined, filed out the door, down the hall, down the industrial-looking staircase that opened directly backstage. The area behind the stage was dimly lit and surprisingly large, cluttered with a variety of strange-to-me equipment, desks and control panels, ropes and pulleys. There was no time to investigate—we slipped directly through doors that seemed to be thirty feet tall and onto the stage. My footsteps echoed across the golden oak sprung stage floor as I followed the singers to my seat. Five rows of black-cushioned, armless chairs sat on risers on the stage, twenty chairs to a row. In front of these were a conductor's podium, a scattering of chairs and music stands for the thirty-piece orchestra, and on the left side of the stage three large kettle drums and an organ.

Once seated, I looked around in awe. Ornate walls of ivory and gold were everywhere, towering around the forty-foot by eighty-foot Perelman Stage some forty feet into the air, supporting a domed ceiling. In front of us was the Stern Auditorium, its famous plush red upholstered seats and vast tiers of ornate carved balconies stair-stepping into a seeming infinity. I was humbled. How was I worthy to be here? Dress rehearsal was a daze.

That evening, with little time for small talk, nine of the ten of us from the Downers Grove Choral Society gathered back in the dressing room for a few moments. One alto, who was often late, would eventually show up, we trusted. After a few nervous words, we gathered into our respective vocal sections to warm up and listen to a brief pep talk from our director.

I slipped a XyliMelt into my mouth and attached the lozenge to my lower gum, where it would be held while singing. I hoped it would be enough to keep my mouth moist and prevent a bout of uncontrollable coughing on stage. I also feared it might come loose and I would choke on it.

We stood in the large room gathered around our director, David Puderbaugh. If he was nervous like the rest of us, he didn't show it. He seemed confident and professional, a forty-ish, slim, balding man with a neatly trimmed short beard and mustache, wearing a crisp black tuxedo with a white embroidered vest and white silk tie.

I kept glancing toward the door, worried that the missing alto wouldn't make it this time after all. Then she pushed her way to her place next to me, looking rushed and slightly embarrassed. I didn't say a word.

Conductor Puderbaugh paused, looked in her direction, then addressed our group. He led us through a ten-minute warm-up, then smiled at us broadly.

"You've got this," he said. "You've done all that needs to be done. Now go make music."

Anyone who has sung with a classical choir knows that on stage during a performance, a singer has little time to think about anything except singing. Concentration on the complexities of a piece such as the *Mariazeller Mass*

has to be absolute.

The beauty of a choral work is marked by its unity and precision. The worst thing a singer can do in a chorus is stand out from other singers by beginning before the chorus does, holding a note longer than the chorus, or singing over the chorus. This requires precise timing, counting every beat in every measure, even those measures in which you don't sing. And to complicate matters further, the conductor is always altering the tempo, so, without missing a single beat, you must change instantly to his baton.

We work this out in rehearsal, yet in performance all bets are off. The conductor, as the music speaks to him, improvises on the spot to bring out the best interpretation of the music. If all a singer had to do was learn the melodies and when to sing loud or soft, choral singing would be easy. Without precise timing, the performance becomes a train wreck, and the music grinds to a halt. A do-over, especially in so revered a concert hall, would be hugely embarrassing.

Would this evening end for me in disgrace or triumph?

Tonight, the *Kyrie* begins hushed, pianissimo, but by the third measure swells to forte. I sing louder but hold back my full voice to avoid straining. The other altos will carry the part in the louder passages. The soprano soloist picks up in the ninth measure, switching from 4/4 to 3/4 time and a lively tempo. While the chorus is silent, I glance toward Chris and Bob in the second balcony. Neither of them cares for classical music. I wonder if they're impressed. I hope they are.

Twelve measures later the chorus resumes in forte. I count the measures with my right toes. We're not supposed to toe-tap, but I do it inconspicuously. I'm not supposed to bury my head in my music either—I should lift my head and watch the conductor. I do my best to keep my eyes up, but I check the music frequently so I don't lose my place.

The *Kyrie*, difficult but not especially challenging, ends after about eight minutes. I haven't missed a note, nor have I screeched. I give a relieved sigh and glance to the second tier where Chris and Bob are seated. Just a glance, as the conductor's baton is up again, and he is waiting for all eyes to be on him before he gives the downbeat for the *Gloria*. And it comes!

This is going to be harder. The *Gloria* is long, about ten minutes, with only a two-minute soprano solo near the beginning. The piece is dramatic and lively, and it ends with a fugue. Fugues are probably the most difficult passages for choruses to sing. A phrase is introduced by one part, and then successively each part—soprano, alto, tenor, and bass—takes up the phrase, altering each repeat with variations, and interweaving the melodies with the other parts. Somehow, we all have to end up on the right chord at exactly the same time. The fugue in the *Gloria* is long, about three minutes, and difficult. In rehearsal we "derailed" multiple times, requiring many repeats.

We are singing in Latin. We must pronounce the unfamiliar words correctly, using the vowels the conductor prefers, being careful that consonants are clear but not too hard or too soft, which would make the words seem silly to the ear—and all one hundred singers must stop the sound at exactly the same moment, especially consonants like "t," otherwise the audience hears a stutter!

It's not only about fast or slow, loud or soft, the right pronunciation of the words, and how long to hold the notes. It's also about the mood, be it awed, dramatic, joyful, or lively. So I can understand the meaning and emotion of the text, I translate the Latin to English in my head.

The chorus begins joyously: "*Gloria in excelsis Deo, et in terra pax…* Glory to God in the highest, and peace on earth…"

My heart swells! I'm captured by the joy of the music. Tears form, but I blink them away so I can see my score clearly and lift my voice. The altos, my section, begin the fugue. "*Amen,*" over and over, in a variety of melodic phrases by each separate part, rising in volume and tempo to the climactic and definitive final note. On the high notes, my swollen throat tightens and no sound comes out. It's mildly painful, but I need not have worried. I'm not alone, but part of a team, and each of us has truly done our part.

The phrases are long. We can't all breathe at the same time, or the audience would hear a mass gasp. The conductor has had us mark where we can safely—and quietly—breathe, but there are places we must sneak breaths where we can, not all at the same time.

The *Credo* is next, at twelve minutes the longest piece in the Mass, which also ends with a three-minute fugue. It begins dramatically, with joyful phrases declaring what we believe: "*Credo in unum Deum*, I believe in one God…."

This time the basses lead the fugue. The phrases are lively, like dancing, and so catchy that we have had less trouble learning the parts, and in fact they have become earworms, repeating in our heads for days now. This is perhaps our favorite part of the Mass. "*Et vitam venturi saeculi*…for the life of the world to come!" This phrase is repeated over and over. The crispness of the Latin words seems to add life to the rapid, dancing notes as they are brought out by first one part and then another.

After the soft, melodic *Sanctus*—"Holy Lord God"—and the lyrical *Benedictus*—"Blessed is He"—we have arrived at the last work, the *Agnus Dei*, or Lamb of God. The most challenging fugue in the Mass.

I am worried now. My voice is tired, taut, and strained, but still producing the right sounds, if a bit more weakly. Of more concern is my mouth dryness. A mis-swallow or an ill-advised sudden breath of air hitting the back of my throat—or absolutely no reason at all—would set me into an uncontrollable coughing spell. If that happened, I would have to drop down behind the other singers and hope I could stifle enough of the sound to save the performance and the recording that was being made. I couldn't ruin the concert for everyone!

To top it off, I have never gotten through this fugue without losing my place. Yes, I can fake it, move my mouth and emit no sound, and let the chorus fill in for me. But this is my one shot at being able to brag that I sang at Carnegie Hall and take pride in what I did here. Maybe if those around me lose their place, I can be the one who helps them find it. But only if I don't miss a note.

This fugue, which is not unusual for ending fugues, is full of runs, or melismas. These are strings of notes that are sung on a single syllable but have very short values. They are combinations of sixteenth notes (four notes to a single beat), eighth notes, and other values, all strung together and sung extremely rapidly. A singer must not only arrive at the right pitch but hold the note for an extremely short time, but the *correct* short time, and do this while everyone around her is singing something else at the *same* time. The combinations required in a particular piece make it hard, and this fugue, called the "*Dona nobis pacem*, or "grant us peace," is hard! At least, it's hard for me.

I would not be able to look up from my music to get through this part. Fortunately, I had trained myself to catch the movements of the conductor from a corner of my eye and learned to make my voice respond in an instant to what my ears pick up around me. If the audience doesn't see my eyes, well, it will have to be for the four minutes the fugue lasts! Photos of the concert will show me looking down, not into the camera, but I'm resigned to that.

I plunge into the fugue, at full voice now, since it makes no difference if I have any voice left after this.

I nail it! I don't make a single error!

The audience jumps to their feet, applauding and cheering wildly. I meet the eyes of Chris and Bob and smile broadly. For this I had come. The peak of my singing career, the culmination of my struggle, my triumph over tongue cancer and other demons, ended in success.

What I had been through with cancer prior to this day made the experience that much more precious.

I sang at Carnegie Hall!

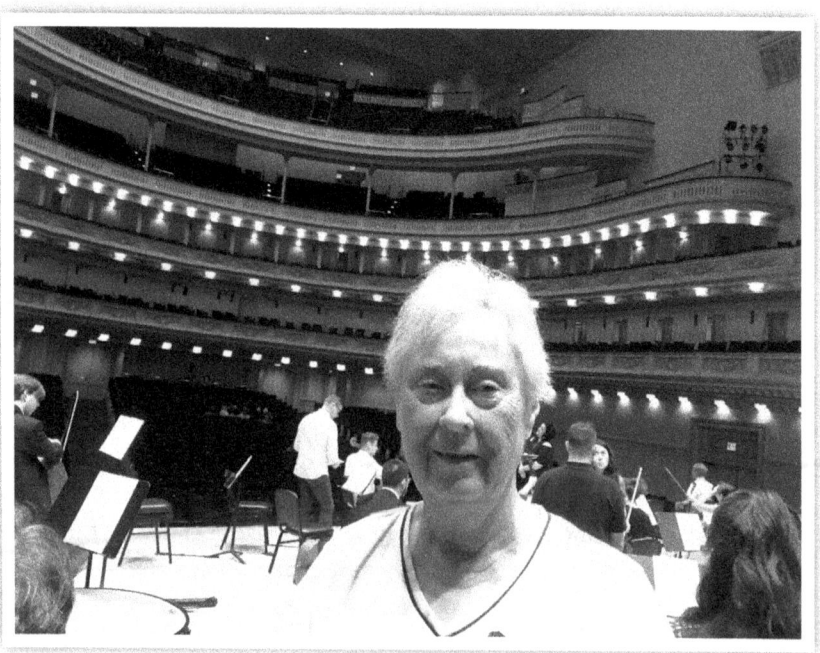

Me at Carnegie Hall dress rehearsal.

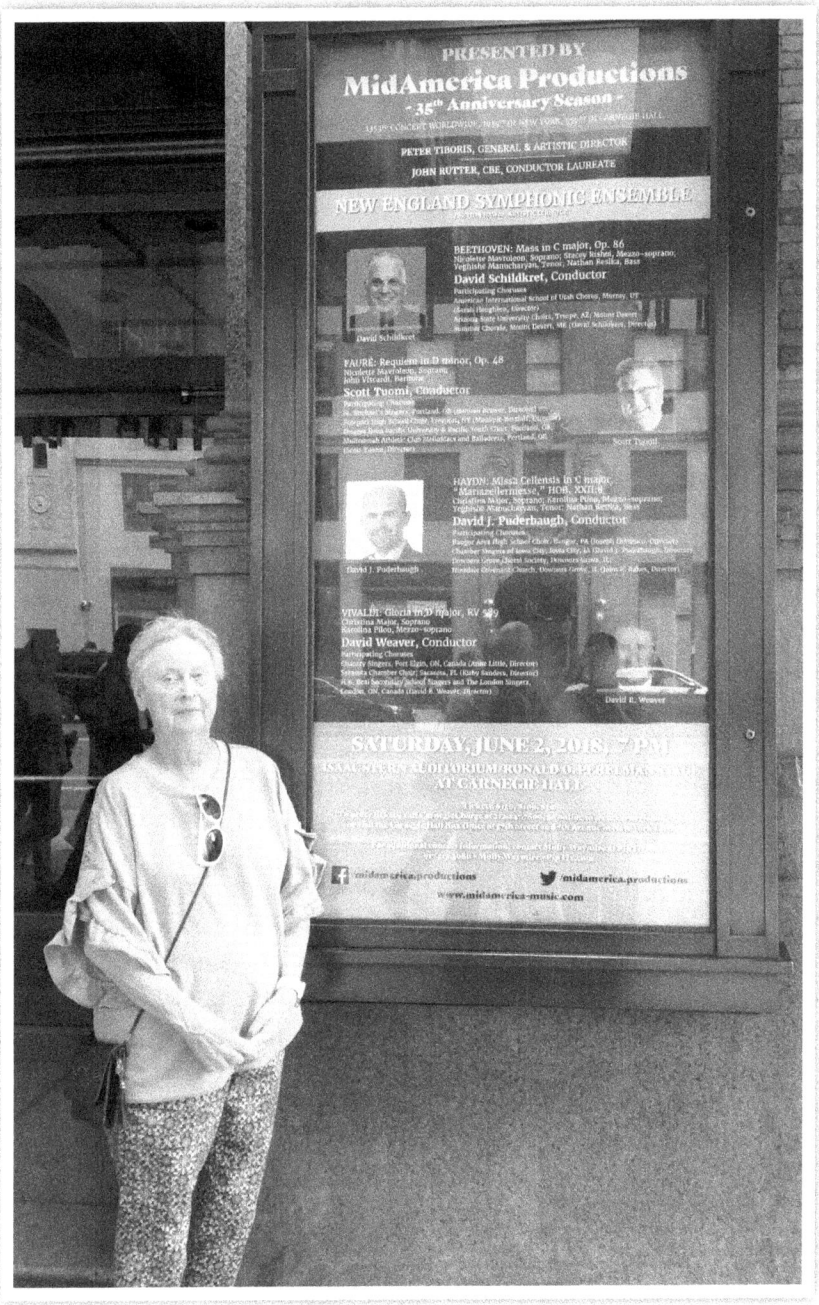

Me at Carnegie Hall Billboard.

CHAPTER 46
Recovered, but It's Not Over: Lymphedema
June 2018

"The treatment did what it was supposed to do with no surprises after, and you can't always count on that until you do it. Your care was very good. I was impressed with your follow-up, especially your ENT." - Dolly, daughter-in-law

"I was surprised by how much coughing was associated with your recovery, the damage done by radiation." - John, son

Singing in Carnegie Hall created memories of a lifetime. After the concert, Bob, Dolly, and Mia joined Chris and me for sightseeing in New York City. As expected, it was hard to find restaurants that offered good choices for me, but we got through it. A few high points were walking in Central Park and across Brooklyn Bridge (slowly!), the Staten Island Ferry ride, and the visit to the site of 9/11.

While we were in New York, swelling and pressure in my neck and throat became increasingly troublesome. The swelling had begun shortly before we traveled to Carnegie, but I hadn't wanted to jeopardize our plans for the trip, so I didn't do anything about it before we left home.

I knew the cause of the swelling. Three months after my radiation sessions finished, Dr. Thomas told me I had developed lymphedema. Fluid was pooling in my neck, causing pressure against my throat. If I did nothing

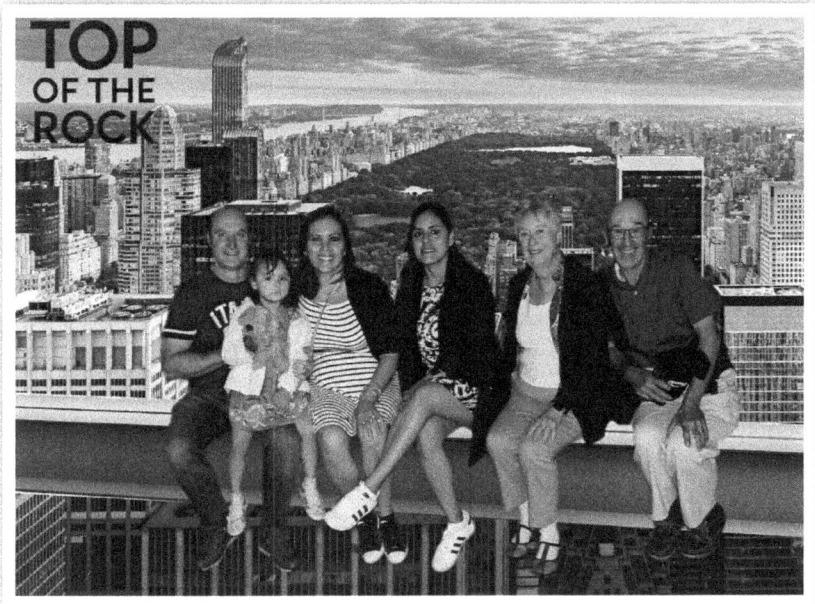

Bob, Mia, Dolly, Jenny (Nanny), me, and Chris touring New York City.

to control lymphedema, it could become permanent.

I had few, if any, lymph nodes in my neck after radiation. This was permanent. The nodes had been infiltrated by my cancer, had been destroyed by radiation, and would not return. I was dependent on remaining lymph vessels in other parts of my body to clear fluid from my neck, and those wouldn't work as efficiently.

Lymph is a liquid that seeps out of thin blood vessels into soft tissues in parts of the body. Normally it will be collected by lymph vessels that carry it to lymph nodes, which then return the liquid to the bloodstream.

Because the lymph nodes in my neck had been destroyed, this process was interrupted. The fluid in my neck can't return to the bloodstream and collects in the soft tissues of my neck and especially below my jaw and around my voice box.

The tightness in my throat got worse and worse while we were in New York, to the point that when I looked in the mirror it seemed to me as if I had a tennis ball where my Adam's apple would be. I started to imagine once again pressure in my neck cutting off my airway and being unable to breathe. I would have to do something about it as soon as we returned.

So I was back at Rush again, once a week this time, for occupational therapy to learn how to reduce the fluid accumulation.

The therapist told me that I had to learn to move the fluid from my neck manually. She taught me how to massage my neck and gave me new exercises to do at home for twenty minutes twice a day. I also wore an elastic support around my neck, jaw, and head for four hours a day. The appliance was skin-colored, but it was an ugly thing that I was embarrassed to wear in public.

While learning the massage techniques, I observed myself in a mirror to be sure I was doing them right. Chris found me standing in front of the bathroom sink.

"Do you think that's doing you any good?" he asked, watching me from the doorway.

"Some, I guess," I said, gently stroking my neck. "Already I don't feel like my throat is closing shut anymore. I can swallow better. But I hate this lump." I poked at my voice box, then I grabbed a mass of tissue under my chin between my thumb and forefinger.

"And if this sac gets any bigger, I'll look like a turkey."

"The gift that keeps on giving, isn't that what Dr. Layan said? I guess you'd better keep up the therapy then." He stepped away from the doorway, then turned back and said, "Gobble, gobble."

Neck massages would keep the accumulation from increasing and lessen the danger that the accumulation itself would harden and become permanent. "Late effects," they're called, lymphedema and jaw muscle problems.

Four months after completing cancer treatment, seven months after my diagnosis, much of my life was still overshadowed by cancer. Only a little of my sense of taste had returned, and although I was eating fairly well, I still didn't enjoy food. I had to be careful with each swallow I took, and I had to cut food like burgers with a knife and fork instead of biting because I couldn't open my jaw wide enough.

In addition to neck massages, I continued speech therapy exercises for my jaw muscles and swallowing function. I walked every day. Due to radiation, I have a lifelong risk of cavities in my teeth and bone loss in my jaw. Brushing teeth and scraping tongue, rinsing, fluoride treatments—I did all these multiple times daily too, and they all took time.

I was tired of living that way and I would have much preferred to do nothing. The exercises and dental routines—about two hours daily—took much less time, though, than the full days of medical activities months before. So I had much of my day back for other things.

Also, on the plus side, my skin had healed, except that my neck was sensitive to touch due to nerve damage. I had to avoid exposing my skin to the sun, probably for life. I rarely had nausea or pain anymore, except for mild throat irritation. I saw Dr. Thomas, Dr. Fidler, and Dr. Layan regularly, along with my speech and occupational therapists. I no longer saw a dietitian.

By July, my energy was almost all back. I resumed a full schedule of board meetings and volunteer activities. I rarely napped, I got up and retired at a reasonable hour, and I fell asleep in front of the TV—like I did pre-cancer, but without crashing! At last, I no longer felt sick or drained when I woke up.

I couldn't return to personal appearances and speaking engagements yet. After about ten minutes of using my voice, my mouth would start to feel like it was sticking together, it became difficult to move my tongue, and my voice got weak and raspy. Even worse, I feared the dryness would trigger a violent coughing spell, which happened at home up to a couple of times a day if I wasn't careful speaking or swallowing, and sometimes even when I was careful. I didn't want to have such a spell on the speaker's stand. It would be hugely embarrassing to be coughing and unable to speak for ten minutes or longer, doubled over, gasping, and possibly losing bladder control. I couldn't take that risk.

Instead, I did a few exhibits, signings, book clubs, etc. My pace was slower than before, but when I got tired, I stopped. I didn't allow myself to get pressured into doing too much too soon—although that was against my nature! I liked to be busy and hated to say no.

I picked up where I left off writing *The Mystery at Mount Forest Island*, hoping to finish it before the end of the year.

On July 20 Chris and I drove to Fort Wayne for Mia's third birthday. We arrived late Friday for the party that was scheduled for Saturday afternoon. There would be about forty people, including all our family, Dolly's mother who was visiting from her home in Lima, Peru, and a multitude of friends. A wood-fired pizza oven would provide catering for the event.

The weather was perfect, and we ate in the yard and swam in the pool between catching up with friends. I didn't swim while the guests were present, because my old bathing suits were much too large and hung on me revealingly and embarrassingly. But I'm proud to say I was able to help with decorations, preparing appetizers, and clean-up. My favorite photo captured Chris and I hugging Mia in front of a serving table and a collection of balloons that included a huge gold number three and a unicorn with a pink mane.

On the way home from Fort Wayne, Chris and I stopped at a discount mall in Michigan City, and I indulged in what I call "shameless shopping." After dropping three sizes, Dolly had already taken me shopping to my favorite clothing stores and bought me new clothes. I intended to buy a few odds and ends. We hit sales though, and I'm a sucker for sales. I won't tell you how much I bought; it was great stuff but more than I needed. Way more. I was disgusted that I had given in to such temptation, but at the same time part of me thought I deserved a reward after my recent struggles.

This short trip sticks in my mind as being a milestone to mark my recovery. At last, I was able to spend most of my time without thinking about cancer. I could even say that life was good once again.

I began to think of my cancer as being in the past. I had lost my sense of taste and my appetite for the better part of a year with slow improvement. I had had a sore throat from beginning to end, but it was never awful. I suffered burns and other painful skin conditions and extreme fatigue. Some conditions could still occur, but I began to think the worst was over at last.

The experience—and it wasn't over yet—had been tough in ways I never imagined but easy in some of the ways I feared. It brought the unexpected from the very beginning and was still bringing surprises. It's anyone's best guess whether it was strength or bullheadedness that got me through.

Cancer leaves you with new norms. Every time you think you have mastered life again, something new comes up. But you've strengthened your resilience by facing cancer, the demon has been put in his place, and these new problems by comparison are more like inconveniences than life-threatening. You've proved you were up to it and won the battle.

Here's a shout-out from the woman who survived tongue cancer and ended up singing in Carnegie Hall!

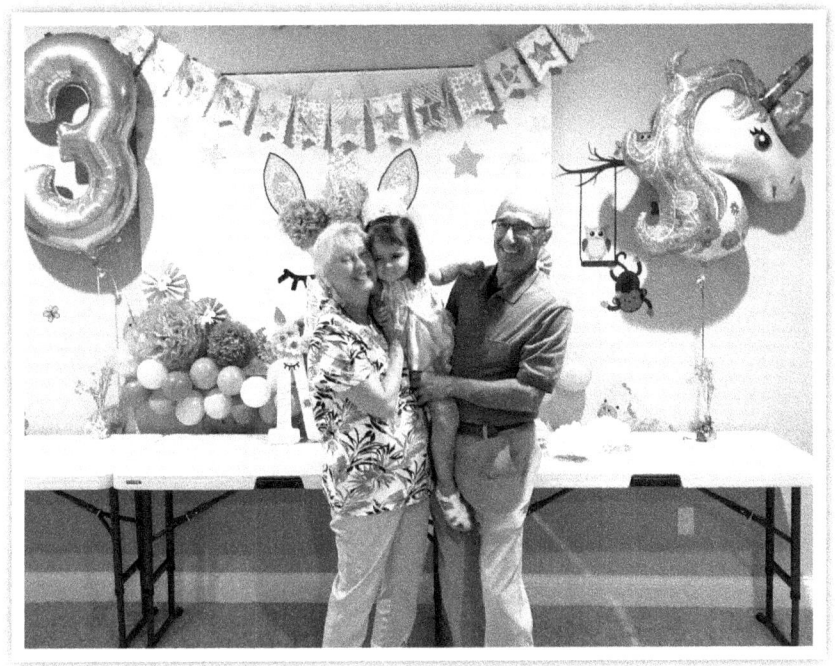

Chris and me with Mia on her third birthday

CHAPTER 47

What About Now? Late Effects
August 2023

"It's five years and you're still here. - John, son

"My strongest memory is when you were here for Thanksgiving and you said, 'I've got this lump.'" - Bob, son

Three months after we returned from New York, Chris had a stroke and was found to suffer from atrial fibrillation. Then, as soon as he regained his health, my friend Dorothy, who had sent me the prayer box and been such a support through my illness and Chris's hospitalization, died from brain cancer in January 2019.

These tragedies hit me hard. These two people had been instrumental in my successful triumph over cancer, and I wanted to support them as they had supported me. It was impossible to do as much as I wanted for both of them at the same time.

Eventually the string of catastrophes ended. I finished and released the book I'd had to set aside, *The Mystery at Mount Forest Island*, in April of 2020, shortly after COVID stopped all personal appearances. I learned to use Zoom and kept up with author events on that platform, but struggled to get the hang of promoting book sales remotely.

Meanwhile, I kept my cancer surveillance follow-up appointments. First monthly, then bimonthly, then quarterly, then semi-annual laryngoscopies were performed, and I remained NED—no evidence of disease.

Fortunately, most of my sense of taste returned and after a year I was able to enjoy food again. Now when I first put food in my mouth, it tastes pretty much as I remember it, but after a few bites the intensity of the flavor fades. The taste isn't unpleasant but isn't as rich as those first bites. That's acceptable to me.

I got used to a dry mouth and learned to swallow carefully. Food still sticks now and then, and I still have coughing attacks occasionally, but I accept these inconveniences. I can talk in public again if I keep water at hand and take brief pauses when needed. My voice is strained afterward but recovers nicely the next day.

By early 2022 I was told that, although the magic five-year mark that usually denotes a cancer survivor would not arrive until March of 2023, recurrence of my cancer was highly unlikely. Even if cancer was found again, it would be considered to be new, not from my original tongue cancer.

It wasn't long after remission that I started to have some of those "late-effect" conditions I had been warned about. I did, as expected, have a lot of radiation changes. The symptoms I have consist of swelling and pressure in my throat and occasional difficulty swallowing. I wish I didn't have these symptoms, but I can live with them. That's good because I have to do just that.

About nine months after finishing treatment, my thyroid hormone levels dropped below normal. Most patients with radiation to the neck will suffer some damage to their thyroid glands. I have no symptoms at all, and this condition, fortunately, was easily corrected with a prescription for a low dose of Synthroid. My blood tests have stayed normal on this medication.

More than two years after cancer diagnosis, I started to have pain in my jaw. I was told that my symptoms were caused by fibrosis, or scar tissue, due to radiation. Over time, I got used to eating with some jaw discomfort, but I still must stop chewing and rest my jaw during meals.

My hard-to-control coughing spasms continued. I was told this was because radiation had reduced the normal sensation at the back of my throat. This allows liquids to trickle, solids to irritate. Spurts of saliva, or even air or absolutely nothing can cause a cough. There is little to be done other than to learn avoidance techniques through experience.

A year later I started having dental problems. Dental decay, gum, and jaw disease are among the most common side effects of radiation to the head. Two rear teeth in my upper jaw broke off at the gumline, leaving only roots, and extractions were recommended. However, I had two problems that made extractions inadvisable. Because I have osteopenia, I had an infusion to treat that condition, and that medication interferes with bone healing. Secondarily, radiation made extraction inadvisable because of increased risk of osteonecrosis of the jaw.

I have good dental hygiene and I see my dentist regularly and follow his instructions. I *don't* have osteonecrosis, but when I developed the broken teeth, the *risk of getting* osteonecrosis was a real eye-opener for me.

Osteopenia, which I do have, means that my bones have less than the desired amount of calcium, and therefore are weaker. It's very common, especially for older, fair-skinned women like me, and has nothing to do with my radiation. But if it isn't treated, it's likely to develop into osteoporosis, which means that bones become brittle and break easily. A simple fall can result in life-changing fractures.

Osteonecrosis is even more serious. It means that the blood supply to the bone is cut off and the bone dies. Yes, despite its hardness, bone is *living* tissue. Osteonecrosis would cause pain and possible destruction of the bone, and it's hard to treat, possibly requiring surgery and, due to the area in question for me, an artificial jaw implant.

The jaw is particularly susceptible to osteonecrosis because the bone is more easily exposed there, covered by only a thin layer of tissue. My radiation to the jaw is likely to have weakened the bone to some extent.

With both conditions, those caused by radiation and the interference with healing from my infusion, I had increased risk that extracting the teeth could cause the bone in my jaw to die.

My medical doctors advised me to avoid extractions unless there was no other option. This didn't mean that extractions *would* cause osteonecrosis, but that there was increased risk. Nor was it likely to be a life-threatening condition—only a painful and possibly disfiguring condition.

I didn't like those odds. We decided to leave the roots of the broken teeth in place and to replace the lost chewing area with a partial denture.

That solution wasn't ideal, but it's working.

At the end of 2022, four years post cancer diagnosis, I developed a burning sensation in my left external ear. Over time the sensation traveled down the left side of my neck and eventually to the front of my neck. It felt like mild sunburn, but without redness or rash. I saw my internist, my ENT, and a neurologist. Examinations by all three doctors and work-up including an MRI of my neck did not show a cause for the problem. There was no new cancer, and the likely diagnosis was that the problem was another side effect, resulting from radiation damage internally and to the nerve endings in my skin.

I saw a speech therapist again to access the level of fibrosis and lymphedema more than five years after I finished radiation. She showed me pictures from my laryngoscopies so I could understand how internal pressure from radiation damage was affecting my ability to swallow. I saw how the space above my epiglottis had shrunk, forming an area where food collected.

Radiation changes were also contributing to lymphedema. The physical therapy I'd had for lymphedema during my recovery period had reduced it considerably, so I had gotten lazy about doing the daily massages I'd been taught. Five years later I realized I shouldn't have stopped this regime. The symptoms I was having were a new presentation of the same condition.

Up to seventy-five percent of patients who have the sort of radiation I had experience some level of lymphedema, often many years later.

But how bad was mine? What could I do about it? How does lymphedema relate to radiation fibrosis? To the nerve endings in the skin of my neck and ears?

Initially my lymphedema was in the area just under my skin, or external lymphedema. Now the radiation damage was deeper, or internal. The damage was early, but it decreased the efficiency of swallowing, my neck muscles were unusually tight, and the skin of my neck and ears were uncomfortable with a pins-and-needles sensation. I didn't want this to get worse and lead to bigger problems.

The idea was to control the formation of more fibrosis by controlling the lymphedema, and that was done by better massage techniques. I also had to resume swallowing and jaw-stretching exercises.

Slowly the burning faded, but my external ears and neck remain numb until this day. This is another annoyance I live with. It's uncomfortable when clothing touches my neck or my ears, when I wear glasses, or when I rest my head on either side. I don't like the discomfort, the time-consuming routines, and the reminders that cancer could be lurking nearby. But it's better than having cancer.

These realizations made me grateful once again that I had opted for the more targeted course of radiation my doctors had offered. The late effects would likely have been considerably worse with standard therapy.

It may seem that I have gone on overly long about these late effects. I do so because I don't want to leave a false impression that surviving cancer is happy-ever-after. Cancer will continue to present problems and worries. And yet, life after cancer is a good life. I have reached the "cure date." I have a few problems that are probably permanent, but in the large picture they are annoying more than life-threatening.

Although I'd much prefer not to have all these side effects, they have all been manageable. They don't stop me from doing the things I want to do. Life's a little harder, but when is life always easy?

Probably the biggest effect on my life is one of a sense of underlying worry. Once you have cancer, you know what the experience is like, and you don't want to go back there. What a "normal" person would do when a new symptom occurs is chalk it up to aging or wait patiently to see if it goes away. My first reaction is, *is this cancer again?* I try to remain calm and patient, but there's that underlying fear in my subconscious, that sinking in my gut, that mild nausea that remains until cancer is excluded.

Although I now see most of my doctors only every six months, there are a lot of doctors to see. I have an internist, oncologist, radiation oncologist, otolaryngologist, dermatologist, rheumatologist, neurologist, cardiologist, ophthalmologist, thoracic surgeon, dentist, oral surgeon, and occupational, speech, and physical therapists. This is my long-term team.

Sadly, I had to give up singing. I used to be an alto, but now I find it difficult to reach notes even in the tenor range. I could make the change and sing as a tenor, but I'm still subject to sudden coughing spells and times when I emit a screech or my throat freezes and no sound at all comes out. Straining to reach a note actually causes pain now that radiates up both sides of my neck into my head. Due to pressures in my throat from radiation fibrosis, the muscles in my neck spasm when they are engaged to reach high notes.

I found after trying a couple of concerts that it was too difficult to perform on stage, where my voice is strained over a long period of time in ways that can cause a coughing spell. Performing in front of an audience is also very uncomfortable. On stage, with exact timing and specific raising and lowering of my voice, I cannot manage the breaks, swallows, and water I take to alleviate these conditions. I've considered rehearsing with the group just for the joy of group singing, with no intent of performing in concert. I may decide to do that at some future time.

Not being able to sing left a vacuum in my life, but I had to make a choice between writing engagements and singing engagements, as I didn't have enough time to do justice to both.

But I had the satisfaction of knowing that at Carnegie Hall I had ended my career as a singer on a high note!

I also travel less than I'd like, but that decision is more because of fear than inability. My worry button is pushed when I consider traveling away from my doctors where we can get the level of medical care Chris and I are accustomed to. The incurable worrier that I am.

And so, I have survived cancer and life moves on to other things. I can do whatever is important to me, and I get much pleasure from my family, my friends, and my writing career. I have been fortunate in that I had such good medical care, but I also had strong support from my family and friends, and I worked hard myself. I've had to make compromises, but they aren't big compromises.

Perhaps I've finally found "my time."

EPILOGUE
September 24, 2023

After releasing *The Mystery at Mount Forest Island* in 2020, I began work on a memoir. Knowing both the medical side and the patient side, and how to describe both to readers, made me an ideal person to tell my story. I knew I had helped those who had read my blog, and I felt I owed it to other cancer patients to create a work to help them and their families demystify cancer through my experience.

After beginning the memoir, I struggled. I'm a novelist, so telling the experience through my series character seemed more comfortable to me. I wrote a novel instead.

In late 2022 I published my fourth book, *The Miracle at Assisi Hill*. In this story, my main character is recovering from tongue cancer. I put her in a religious context so she could describe the traumas of her medical experience, the effects it had on her life, and her relationship with God. When things seem impossible, she meets a woman from heaven who visits Earth to help her through. The heavenly visitor is based on the life of a real woman, the Venerable Mother Mary Theresa Dudzik, who is destined to be a saint one day.

In the story, the two women, one on Earth and one in heaven, develop a dependency on each other, immersing them both in the problems each faced individually. As I studied Mother Theresa's story, she affected me deeply. I envied her great compassion, her ability to keep going no matter how hard life got, how she never felt sorry for herself or made excuses, how she always put others ahead of herself, and her heroic virtue.

I met Sister Jeanne Marie in April of 2021 when I visited the Mother Theresa Museum. Venerable Mother Mary Theresa Dudzik founded the Franciscan Sisters of Chicago and built Chicago's first home for the poor and elderly, which opened in 1898. Her sarcophagus and remains reside in the chapel of Our Lady of Victory Convent in Lemont today.

Sister Jeanne Marie Toriskie was the Promoter for Mother Theresa's

STAYING ALIVE IS A LOT OF WORK: ME AND MY CANCER

Cause for Sainthood. Sister Jeanne was friendly and outgoing. She seemed to enjoy answering all my questions and was pleased with my interest and the idea of featuring Mother Theresa in my book. From photos I had seen online, I knew that this order of nuns no longer wore habits. Sister, a tall woman who appeared to be somewhat younger than me, dressed professionally in a modest skirt, blouse, and jacket, her short red hair uncovered by a veil or any headwear.

We liked each other right away, and by the end of the interview an hour and a half later we had become friends. Sister agreed to read and comment on my book. Emails, phone calls, and critiques followed over the next months. The book was published, and we planned to speak together about Mother Theresa to a variety of audiences.

A few days before our first program scheduled at the Lemont Library, Sister Jeanne and I met in her office to go over details of the talk we planned to give. But I had new medical concerns that could affect other programs we planned, and I knew she would want to pray for me.

After five years free of cancer, I had suddenly begun to feel generally unwell and excessively tired, lightheaded, and a little nauseous. The combination of symptoms was concerning.

Heart disease had always frightened me even more than cancer. I knew heart disease could be deadly without warning, and I feared sudden death. A lifelong control freak, I feared dying without being able to prepare. Cancer at least allows one time to identify important matters and get them done.

Once again, I found myself wondering when my life would become my own with no other responsibilities. When could I give up being sick and taking care of others and let someone else take the lead? I was eighty years old. I was tired. Wasn't it time for me to be the child, to let someone else be the boss?

I had extensive work-up that included cardiac studies. The results came back as expected for my age, a little irregular, but nothing that needed treatment, medication, or behavior changes. Keep doing what I had been doing, I was told. Consider yourself healthy. But I didn't feel healthy.

Then an incidental finding appeared on a CT of my chest that was done as part of my stress cardiogram. A nodule that had been in my chest and stable for several years had grown since the previous surveillance scan two years ago. It now looked suspicious for cancer and the radiologist recommended a biopsy.

Oh no, not again.

I'd been here before. Deja vu all over again, as they say. A repeat performance. I got rid of cancer, but cancer may not be finished with me yet. *May not be.*

I could go into denial again, but this time I knew two things: One, another battle would be hard, but I had the strength to face it; and two, I had family and friends to help and take some of the responsibility off my shoulders.

Dr. Earvolino referred me to a thoracic surgeon.

The surgeon was kind and clear. He drew a sketch of my lungs on a whiteboard and showed Chris and me exactly where the nodule was.

"Here's what we're looking at," he said, pointing to a little circle just inside my chest wall. "It was in your lung before, but now it has grown just a little bit, and that is concerning. But what is it? It could be a new cancer, or carcinoid. It could be from your tongue cancer. Or it could be benign. The CT doesn't tell us that.

"Normally we would do a biopsy to find out what this is, and once we know we can plan to treat it. The problem is, due to the small size, only .8 cm, and location, we can't do a biopsy."

"So what do we do?" I asked.

"Well, we can just watch it for a while and see if it continues to grow. It's growing very slowly. Or we could take it out, which means a lung resection."

He must have seen the fear in my eyes and continued.

"It's in an easy location for a non-invasive excision. We'd take a small piece of your lung, about the size of a peapod. If all goes well, and we expect it will, you'll only be in the hospital overnight. But you'll be hurting for about a month."

"Does my oncologist know about this? I'm afraid this is metastatic, from my tongue cancer," I said, my mouth even drier than usual.

"I'll reach out to Dr. Fidler. I don't think this is from your prior cancer. It's more likely new, but we can't be sure. Let's do this: let's get a PET scan to see if that tells us any more. The scan will tell us if there's any other cancer too. Talk to Dr. Fidler, and then we'll decide."

The PET scan a week later confirmed the lung nodule that was suspicious for cancer, but nothing more definitive. The uptake was low and there was no cancer found anywhere else in my body. Once again, bad news and good news.

I made an appointment with oncology, Dr. Fidler and a radiation oncologist.

The radiation oncologist told Chris and me they could destroy the nodule with radiation. It would be easy to do, and I would not expect any side effects. It would be gone, and I wouldn't need surgery.

But...

If we destroyed the nodule, we wouldn't know what it was—if it was benign, or a new cancer, or if it was metastatic from my previous cancer. Metastasis was unlikely because a single nodule showed on the PET scan. But the only way to know what it was for sure would be to remove the nodule entirely and send it to pathology.

If the nodule was destroyed by radiation, it would be gone forever. But my future care depended on knowing what the nodule was, and we wouldn't know that. That option didn't seem good to me.

Dr. Fidler joined us, and we talked it over again, reviewing the three options:

- Cut it out. That was the surest way—we would know what it was and have the information needed to treat me appropriately afterward. But surgery is always a risk, especially at my age, and it would be painful with a four- to six-week recovery. I no longer fooled myself by thinking it would be easier for me. I knew the doctors were right.

- Destroy it. Easy, not painful. But we wouldn't know what it was in order to plan treatment afterward.

- Wait and watch.

What to do? Bob and Dolly wanted me to avoid surgery if possible, but would support me in whatever decision I made.

I decided to hope for the best, wait a few months, and then get another CT. All my medical team agreed that waiting would not affect my outcome, due to radiographic evidence of how slowly the nodule was growing.

I hoped I would feel better after the waiting period was up. I clung to the possibility that this time it could really be a false alarm. After all, the doctors hadn't said the diagnosis was definitive, only *suspicious* for cancer. The scan that found my tongue cancer years ago had been more certain. But for me the decision was complicated by the fact that this time I wasn't feeling generally well. I didn't think that was due to a new cancer, but that it would affect any treatment option I chose.

Sister Jeanne and I were sitting at a round table in her office when I told her I might have cancer again. She stood up and walked around the table to hug me.

"Oh my goodness! I'm so sorry. I'll tell the sisters. All of us will pray for you."

"Thank you," I said, moved. The situation felt unreal, as the previous situation had felt unreal almost six years ago.

"What are you going to do?" she asked.

I gave her a half smile. "I'm dithering. It's my new favorite word."

Dithering was the same word I used whenever family and friends asked my decision.

The afternoon of September 24, 2023, Sister Jeanne and I spoke about Mother Theresa at the Lemont Public Library.

I was anxious, not only because of my new lung problem. Would people be interested in a program about a potential Catholic saint at a *public* library? With two of us speaking, would we be able to deliver the program in a reasonable length of time? I had limited my part of the program to fifteen minutes, but I didn't know how long Sister Jeanne's PowerPoint presentation would take.

Our purpose was to educate people who didn't know about Mother Theresa and impress them enough that they would make her a part of their lives, include her in their prayers, and increase the potential of documenting miracles that would result in her sainthood.

When the program was over, Sister and I knew it had been a success, my initial fears groundless. Our audience had been interested, asked good questions, and the discussion after our talk was lively.

Chris helped repack the exhibits and handouts Sister had brought into cases and loaded everything into our cars. Sister looked very tired. I knew by how she was moving that her back was hurting her, so I was not surprised when she picked up her purse, sat in a chair, and asked me to sit beside her.

But she had not made this opportunity because of her back.

"I have something to give you," she said. She reached into her purse and pulled out a small metallic object that looked a bit like a brass chalice, about three inches tall. Glass covered the bowl of the chalice, and seen through the glass inside was a small, embroidered flower. She handed it to me. I stared at it, not understanding.

"It's a relic," Sister said. "The flower is stitched around a piece of Mother Theresa's habit."

I was stunned. I knew relics like this were extremely rare. If anyone had the few relics of Mother Theresa's life that remained, it would be Sister Jeanne. But why would she give it to me?

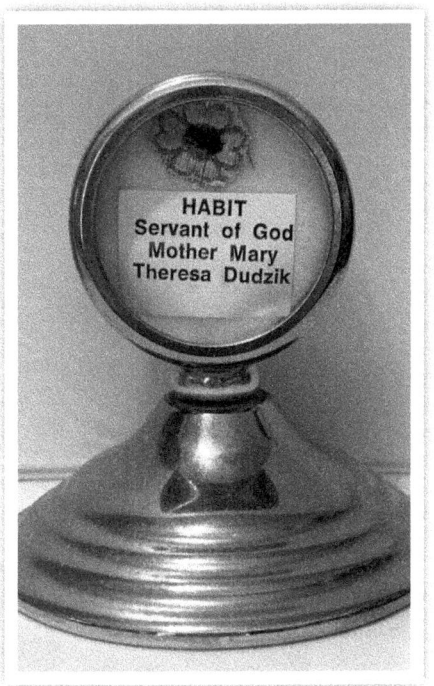

Relic of Venerable Mother Mary Theresa Dudzik

"We only give these to the sisters," she said. "But we regard you as one of us."

Tears came to my eyes, hope and faith came into my heart, but no words came to my lips. "I don't know what to say." Me, the writer, had no words. We stood then and embraced.

"I know your health problems will turn out well," Sister said. "We are all praying for you."

"I think you may be right," I said with a grin. "It seems I've got friends in high places."

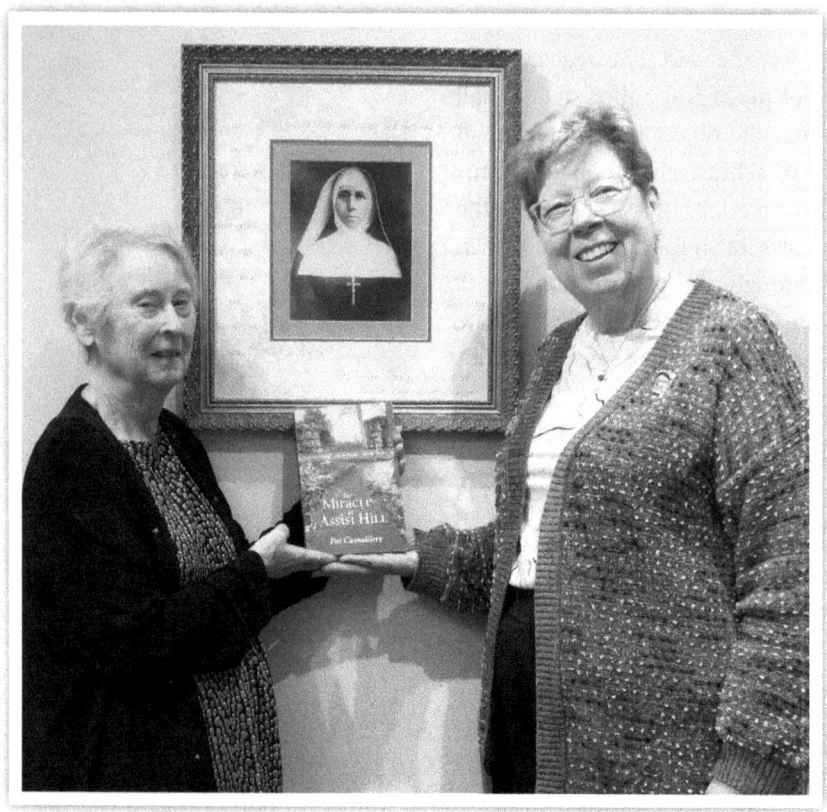

Sister Jeanne Marie and me, with photo of Venerable Mother Mary Theresa Dudzik and copy of my book, The Miracle at Assisi Hill.

APPENDIX I
How Do You Feel Today? Coping with the Emotional Side of Cancer

"I worried about you getting better, about how you would feel afterward, about will you get better. The doctors had confidence and I went along with them. They seemed pretty sure it would work." - Chris, husband.

"I worried about losing you. I hoped you wouldn't get depressed. I worried about how we would handle things, what your wishes would be, and taking care of Chris, if the worst happened. All those thoughts run through your mind." - John, son

"It was shocking, but there was no grief involved because we knew there was optimism." – Bob, son

"I wasn't so much concerned that you would die from the cancer, but I was concerned about the treatment. I think I would have been a more emotional mess." - Clare, daughter-in-law

"We are family. We wanted to help more… When you finish, it is a big relief. We celebrate that it is done." – Dolly, daughter-in-law

One of my writing references is *The Emotion Thesaurus* by Angela Ackerman and Becca Puglisi. The book details some seventy-five emotions. By the time I was into my third month of recovery I think I experienced almost all of them at one time or another.

I'm a writer of fiction—of stories. Perhaps the quote from the writer E. L. Doctorow explains my preference for story over fact: "The historian will tell you what happened. The novelist will tell you what it felt like." This appendix is intended to tell you what it felt like to be a cancer patient.

Emotion is a big part of novel-writing. Fiction, and memoirs too, are popular because they allow readers to place themselves in the story and feel what the character feels. Many think novels convey information more accurately than statements of fact.

I have come to realize that a novel is not a single idea but thousands of ideas that work together. The challenge to us writers is to explore more than one concept or event while keeping the work unified and compelling.

It takes hard work and skill.

As most people would, throughout the course of my illness I experienced a gamut of emotions. I expected that, but I'm a control freak who didn't want to be left an emotional cripple by this disease, so I used a variety of coping mechanisms.

As a result of my upbringing, my emotions have always been conflicted. My mother's image of herself was of an average but intelligent, quiet, and moral woman. True to her Polish heritage, she worked hard and kept her emotions under tight control. She was not a touchy-feely mother. But she was a good mother.

My father, on the other hand, was over-emotional, felt things very deeply, but was embarrassed to show what he was feeling. To do so would have been against his self-image of the happy-go-lucky man in control. This was the man I had to drag sobbing loudly down the aisle when he gave me away at my first wedding.

A product of that conflicting upbringing and genetics, I wanted to give my emotions free reign, but the see-sawing parental experiences in my childhood had instilled in me coping mechanisms for putting a brake on my feelings. My experience with cancer put coping to the test.

In the beginning, I had a tender lump in my neck that I felt sure would go away with an antibiotic. I felt fine, but my doctors told me I wasn't fine—I had cancer. If I didn't fight it, the cancer would win, and I would die. My initial emotional reactions were those of denial, amazement, reluctance, skepticism, surprise, and shock.

This isn't happening. It's a mistake, or a bad dream. I'll wake up and laugh about it.

I couldn't have a life-threatening disease. I don't even want to say the words.

For me, the hardest part, the most stressful part, was making the right decision. Until all decisions were made, my emotions were characterized by fear, anxiety, dread, guilt, nervousness, suspicion, uncertainty, and worry. Most of these emotions should be obvious, especially fear of the unknown course my life had taken so suddenly.

But why guilt, suspicion, and uncertainty? People in my generation grew up with an exaggerated sense of responsibility. I tortured myself with a variety of thoughts:

What did I do to cause this? (Nothing.)

Are those test results right? (They were.)

Surely there's some mix-up! (There wasn't.)

Should I agree to the recommended treatment? (I did, and I think I made the right choice.)

What's going to happen to me? Will I live? I don't want to think about this now! (I have to.)

During that uncertain time, when I couldn't know what was ahead and whether anything was worth doing, I took a mild relaxing medication that calmed me down during waking hours and allowed me to sleep through the night.

After I decided to follow the recommended treatment plan, new emotions set in: acceptance, avoidance, and sadness. I put off thinking about actually having cancer, studied the wealth of information my doctors had given me in a detached way, and didn't do a lot of other research. I wanted to avoid confusion between what I read and what my medical team told me to do. I didn't want to be second-guessing every step of the way. Instead, I engaged myself in a rush of activity.

Okay, I have to do this thing, so I'd better get ready.

I scurried around, getting necessary—and probably some not-really-so-necessary-after-all— tasks done, distracting myself. I was pretty good at that, having practiced other seriously challenging times in the past by simply not allowing myself to think about unpleasantness and throwing myself into activity.

I couldn't avoid thinking about cancer entirely, of course. But rather than let fear take over my life, I set aside specific times when I could be alone to give emotions and fears free reign. Often those moments took the form of conversations with God, which I see as a type of prayer.

I might allow myself to consider what was to come before I got up in the morning, or maybe at bedtime. I might sit in a chapel if that could be arranged, or in a quiet room where I could be sure such private moments wouldn't be interrupted, or, if the weather permitted, walk outside on the block or in my yard.

I planned these sessions carefully. First, I'd select a particular routine task, something like doing laundry or paying bills that kept me busy and occupied my mind without a great deal of thought. Having decided on that task, I'd move to that day's private space.

I'd look at my watch and set a specific amount of time—rarely more than twenty minutes. Then I'd let my thoughts and fears take over. I'd allow myself to put what was bothering me into words, and I'd tell God about it and ask his help. Although I was willing to let myself cry or sob, that never happened. I did get sad and teary-eyed though. When my allotted time was up, I'd permit myself some concluding thoughts. Then I'd turn to that task I had selected ahead of the session to be sure my mind didn't go back to my fears.

I can't say that I got any obvious insights from these sessions, but I do believe there was value in not suppressing my fears entirely. I found that I was calmer and made some decisions that helped me through the course of treatment. I did this throughout treatment and recovery, as often as I needed to, but never more than once a day. I think the experts refer to this technique as compartmentalization.

Routinely my doctors asked if I felt depressed. I often felt dread when I woke up in the morning, but I wouldn't have called that depression. The feeling passed after I got up and began moving through morning routines. I didn't want to worry Chris unnecessarily by discussing that feeling further with my doctors, and he was always in the room with me when the question was asked. So, I just said I got a little down some days, but I was handling it, and left it at that.

When I started treatment, I was determined, confident, defensive, eager, and resigned.

I've made the best decision I can and prepared as well as possible.

This is happening, so there's no use crying about it.

I'm not going to like this (resigned), but the sooner I get started the sooner it will be over (eager).

Life has been tough before and I've gotten through it (determination, confidence).

Don't confuse me—I'll decide who's giving the best advice and follow it my way. (defensive).

Then side effects set in, and I became annoyed, confused, frustrated, insecure, overwhelmed, my thoughts doubtful and conflicted—and surprised again:

I'm doing everything they're telling me to do as well as I can. Why isn't it working better?

It's taking every moment of my day! I can't do it all! Impossible!

Am I doing this right? Did I misunderstand the instructions?

Should I take something for pain, or can I tough it out?

Is this minor pain in my chest an expected side effect? Some other medical issue that needs attention? Or maybe just nothing important?

Should I bother a doctor or nurse with this now or wait it out another day? Maybe I'll be better in the morning...

Am I blowing this out of proportion? After all, everyone says I'm doing so well...

I'm soooooo tired!

When I wasn't at the hospital, I was home with Chris. He sensed when to leave me alone and when I wanted company. I didn't need to be alone for emotional reasons, but because I needed a lot of rest. I was happy to see friends and family but afraid visitors might stay too long and tire me too much.

Later, the side effects got worse, and I started to feel anguish, suffering, disgust, hurt, and irritation.

My whole life is this disease! I'm too busy, too unwell, and I'm tired of it.

What new way am I going to suffer tomorrow, and when is today's pain going to stop?

I look disgusting—no one should be around me. These burns on my neck, my dry and wrinkled skin, the awful flaky patches on my face...Stay home, hide. I don't want people to see me.

My breath must smell like something died in my mouth—probably because something IS dying in my mouth—diseased cells!

Yet:

These physical changes are like wearing a badge of courage. People who see me must know what I'm going through.

I was tired of being asked how I was and making up answers to cover my misery. Of course, I knew people were doing their best to be kind and helpful, but I was frustrated that they couldn't understand how bad off I really was. Then I was angry at myself for criticizing their kind attempts.

Don't tell me what to do! I'm already doing my best.

I'd love it if you brought over dinner and a bottle of wine, but I can't eat anything except oatmeal, I can't drink wine, and you've just made me feel bitter about that, thank you very much!

As I neared the end of treatment, I found perseverance and hope. Yes, the neck pain was worse every day, and I was eating less and less, but that last session was coming up.

I'm almost there! I can do it!

This will all be over and I'll be well again.

I just need to get through a few more...

Then it was over, that last day. I was proud, elated. I wanted to share the feeling, so I bought gifts—gift cards, donuts, books, hand-crocheted items—for doctors and staff members.

I'm all done, I won't be seeing you again, but look how you all helped me get through this, shared my sense of accomplishment. Remember me and how grateful I am to you.

I didn't say any of this, but it's how I felt. I smiled and said, "Thank you," and I hoped they knew I wished I could jump and shout, but that's just not me.

Then I was alone, but not really alone. It wasn't loneliness I felt, but abandonment. Chris, my family, my friends were there—all I had to do was ask. I'd be seeing my team for check-ups, and I could call them anytime. But it's not the same as having a daily chance to ask questions, complain, and brag about accomplishments to people who cared about me.

My biggest letdown, the most emotional time I experienced, was shortly after treatment finished, during recovery. I had fooled myself into thinking, no matter how often I was told otherwise, that now my life would go back to normal. Instead, I was worse than ever. I realized the recovery thing was not going to be so great either. I felt the sickest, and I felt deserted by my medical team, almost to the point of panic at times. Recovery was harder and going to take a lot longer than I wanted to admit to myself, let alone anyone else. I didn't even have the satisfaction of knowing that my cancer was cured yet and wouldn't for a while. Maybe cancer would always be in the background of my life. Disappointment, defeat, sadness, desperation, and impatience set in.

Those feelings were transitory. I soon convinced myself to be positive once again. Recovery was just another hurdle on the way to cure. I was too impatient. My strength came back first, and with it my ability to deal with ongoing side effects.

When the third month of recovery began, I started to pick up pieces of my life. I returned to my writer's groups, board meetings, and volunteer activities on a limited basis. Although eating and skin problems persisted, I grew stronger. My days became longer and more productive.

With longer productive days came a sense of relief and renewed determination. I had been dragging my feet, procrastinating another decision, but I made hotel reservations and bought tickets for a trip to New York with the Downers Grove Choral Society to sing at Carnegie Hall in June. I'd have to do less than I customarily do when traveling, plan fewer activities, and move slowly with plenty of rest between. Eating out would be a challenge. But I wouldn't have the same opportunity again, so I'd make it happen somehow.

Throughout my cancer experience:

I didn't cry. During treatment and recovery, I was focused on doing the best I could to live. I didn't allow myself to break down and sob, although I did get teary-eyed a few times. I can get teary-eyed now when I remember the things I endured and the magnitude of misery I experienced. Part of that emotion is gratitude for having survived.

I never lost my sense of humor. I think I inherited this from my father's wry sense of humor and acerbic wit. Once on a gurney in a hospital elevator while attached to oxygen, he accused the other riders of stealing his air. Like Dad, I joked and poked fun at myself—such as when the blueberries turned my tongue black, and the imaginary shaman who attended my radiation therapy sessions, the Johnny Appleseed guy sowing seeds of disease in my body and being a snake-like superhero.

I remained curious, inquiring how each step in the process was expected to work. Writing my blog helped keep that in the forefront, since I had to understand the process well to write about it.

I felt gratitude for many things: for the fact that my cancer had a high cure rate, that I was surrounded by loving and caring family and friends, that I had access to such skilled medical care—my angels and heroes. Grateful that I had good medical insurance and the best medical care I could find. There were times I was overcome with happiness and love from something done for me, like meaningful cards, messages, or gifts from people I didn't expect. Like the inspiring plaque Sue gave me when my cancer was first diagnosed, and the prayer box Dorothy sent me when I was at a low point in early recovery.

I talked to other cancer patients I saw in the hospital or who contacted me through my blog. Some were having a harder time than I was. I empathized and felt sympathy for them.

Despite all attempts not to overthink my situation, I couldn't stop fear from upsetting me from time to time. Fear was based on things I hoped would *not* happen, rather than things that were happening.

Will it hurt?

Will I have to have surgery?

Will I be disfigured?

Will I ever finish all the books I want to write?

Will I see my two-year-old granddaughter grow up?

Am I going to die?

There were emotions I was expected to feel but did *not* feel.

Anger: It's my nature to deal with problems in order: awareness, anxiety, acceptance, decision, and action. I didn't consciously decide not to be angry about being struck with cancer, it just never happened. Perhaps I was too busy to entertain angry thoughts and emotions. Any anger I had was directed at myself when I thought I'd done something wrong.

Indifference: Indifference can be a coping mechanism. I have always believed that life gives a person good and bad. We enjoy it when the good comes and deal with it when the bad comes. Some might call this indifference, but I call it accepting life.

Resentment, envy, and nostalgia: More coping mechanisms. No matter how much I wished I could enjoy the taste of food again, I didn't feel envious when I saw others eating or dwell with nostalgia on the days I enjoyed food. I only wanted my sense of taste to come back. Who or what would I resent? That would mean attaching blame somewhere, and that didn't make sense to me. And nothing about what was happening made me nostalgic. My positive thoughts were on the future, not the past.

Regret: I didn't find myself regretting past actions. I remained hopeful that I would be allowed time to do things that were important to me.

Throughout my cancer treatment friends and readers complimented me on my courage and positive attitude. I never thought I was doing anything out of the ordinary, except perhaps talking honestly about my experience.

But the bottom line was that I didn't have a choice. If I wanted to survive, I realized that anything less than full cooperation with the program would be harming myself. That's what was really going on in my head. I guess that could be called a positive attitude.

It's human nature to search our souls at such life-changing times, though. I realized I could be a better person than I have been, and I continued to pray that I would come out of this experience as that better person and at peace.

APPENDIX II
Acknowledgements
Angels and Heroes

"The longer you were there, the more confident I became. But I was scared all the time." - Chris, husband

"You went to one of the top hospitals in the country. I thought you were in good hands. And you had Bob and Dolly to provide insight." – John, son

"We had confidence in your care team. Rush is a solid institution." - Bob, son

"I felt confident because you had worked at Rush. If you didn't have the right contacts, you knew people who did." - Clare, daughter-in-law

"I didn't think I had to do much for you, not even as much as I do for some of my patients. It's like doing my work, and I like it. If I have that knowledge, I have to do it. Not everyone is capable of doing certain things, so we all have to use our talents." - Dolly, daughter-in-law

Most of my life I had been in control not only of myself but of family and friends and accepted that role. Throughout my cancer treatment, however, I was dependent on a huge cast of characters: the people who made me well again. I grew fond of them, both as individuals and as part of my medical team.

My life as a cancer patient was filled with Angels and Heroes.

Angel: Someone very good, helpful, or kind. Angels make you smile when you see them. They make your day when you are sad or in pain. They are sweet and help people in need, especially those going through really tough times. The name "Angel" says it all.

Hero: A person who is admired or idealized for courage, outstanding achievements, or noble qualities. A hero knows what needs to be done and does it in a superlative way. Heroes don't think they are doing anything unusual. It's just their nature to be that way.

Today an amazing number of these very special people are employed in healthcare. My family and friends also revealed themselves in a new light.

I feel sad that some patients need to face treatment for cancer without support from family, friends, and excellent medical providers. I've spoken a lot about being a worrier, but I never had to worry about being alone or about the quality of my medical care.

Trust is an essential ingredient to the success of medical treatment. I can't imagine how difficult my life would have been if I didn't trust the people and the institution that helped me cure my cancer.

Some people don't agree with me about teaching hospitals. Typically, these people say, "I want to be close to home," or "You're treated like a number in those big places," or "I want to be seen by doctors, not students." I think these comments are based on misconceptions that don't consider level of care, which in my opinion is the single most important thing for any serious medical condition and especially for cancer patients.

If I were to go to the nearest community hospital, it would take at least twenty minutes from leaving my house to entering the building. If it takes an hour instead, my life is worth an extra forty minutes. Or a little more on those days traffic is bad. I waste more time than that on computer games and watching television.

Individual attention at teaching hospitals has improved greatly in recent years. My care at a university hospital was more personal than what I experienced at the community hospitals my mother preferred. The doctors I saw were warm, caring, and generous with their time. I wonder if that was because at community hospitals doctors must do more themselves, whereas at teaching hospitals residents share the work, leaving my doctor more time to spend on studying my case, making decisions, and talking with me.

Some people don't like talking to students and residents and then answering the same questions for their doctor. I, on the other hand, enjoy talking to students and residents. They're eager to help me and to learn from me. They're not in a hurry and they take as much or little time as I like. Also, daily contact with students and residents keeps staff doctors on their toes: doctors have to stay current to teach. My staff doctors were involved in every step of my treatment and made all major decisions. In addition, if one of my doctors was needed elsewhere, a resident could see me until my doctor arrived, instead of a prolonged wait or rescheduled appointment.

Teaching hospitals generally have the most up-to-date equipment, procedures, and the highest standards. Specialists are available quickly in a vast number of areas that are not found locally. Remember that teaching hospitals see the most difficult cases because challenging patients are sent there when community hospitals cannot provide the care required. This level of quality extends to nursing and other professional staff. Statistics prove that consistently teaching hospitals have the best patient outcomes. Given the choice, why not start there to begin with? In my opinion, these benefits outweigh spending some extra minutes on the road.

For me, an added factor is that, since I had worked at Rush for fifteen years before retirement, it was familiar territory.

I would have made the same decision for many reasons, but the clincher was the availability of research studies. In my case, I would not have been offered the clinical study elsewhere—my research protocol with new, and better, options. Most hospitals that are not affiliated with a medical school don't have the staff support required to offer research studies.

Bottom line, for any important medical issues I want the best care available, not the most convenient. What could be more important than saving me from cancer? I have worked in both community hospital and university hospital settings, and I've seen a real difference in quality of care, attitude, and results. You will find me at teaching hospitals. In my opinion, the high standards that a teaching environment creates ups the chances of finding the right people.

I'm fortunate in that I live in an area where there are many fine teaching hospitals to choose from. I chose Rush because I had worked there for many years and had confidence in the institution and doctors, and because of its excellent outcome ratings in many areas of medicine.

That being said, of course angels and heroes are at all hospitals, and good medical care can be found close to home. I'm looking at a particular area of the country where an urban population makes a difference in choice, and this marketplace may not pertain to other areas.

The point is that when deciding where you will receive treatment for cancer, do your homework. If you have an outstanding medical or cancer center nearby but it's not a teaching hospital, go there. But consider all the options you can, and don't be misguided by inconvenience or false information about teaching hospitals.

Let me tell you about my personal angels and heroes.

Cancer is a battle, but the fight should be fought against the disease, never with the people who are helping you through the battle. My battle was always and only against cancer, and my "team" gave their all to help me fight the fight.

To begin at the top, I was fortunate to have a team of doctors I really trusted, who never made me feel rushed and answered all my questions truthfully without sugarcoating. There were four doctors involved in my care:

Dr. Jennifer Earvolino, my internist, recognized that the tender "lump" on the side of my neck was not a simple swollen gland or other benign growth, but something that needed further investigation. She saw me the same day I called her and contacted my otolaryngologist while I waited in her exam room. Before I left the hospital that day, I had already had the CT scan that diagnosed my cancer. This was not an isolated occurrence, but an example of the personal care and speed with which things can happen in a university setting. I credit her quick recognition of my cancer and actions with saving my life.

Dr. Thomas, my otolaryngologist, greeted me with a cheery smile and asked, "What's happening?" He was always upbeat but honest. He gave me confidence. He told me my disease was not easy to treat, but it had a high success rate for cure. "We have ways to fix this." He fit me in whenever I needed him, even to set my mind at ease. One night he called me from his car at eight in the evening after a long day in surgery. I knew he was watching over me in the background, and I believed that under his care things would turn out well.

Dr. Mary Jo Fidler, my medical oncologist, was a quiet and gentle woman. Her relaxed and confident approach made me comfortable. She patiently listened to my complaints and questions. "Everything tastes the same—BAD!" I ranted once. She knew what I was experiencing—I could feel her sympathy. She is noted nationally for her expertise in the field of oncology. She surely saw many people who had the same problems as me and could quickly recognize anything that didn't go as expected and take steps to fix it. Yet she was a straight shooter. "*Why* aren't you doing your massages?"

Dr. Layan, my radiation oncologist, was young, direct, enthusiastic, and charming. I liked him immensely and immediately, and he never let me down. I could tell he wanted my treatment to be successful. He never seemed rushed and often spent long periods of time with me, but he was interested in my life and activities. He gave me his personal email address and invited me to contact him anytime. The few times I called, he got right back to me. He looked for ways to make me more comfortable when side effects began.

Other team members gave me phone numbers and email addresses to contact for scheduling, urgent requests, and minor questions. This availability at all times was heartening. I didn't take advantage of it often, but just knowing I could provided tremendous relief.

Dr. Gold, a resident in head and neck radiation oncology, saw me routinely before, after, or with my radiation oncologist. He was always available to me. He was also enthusiastic, knowledgeable, and took particular interest in me. It was obvious that he cared about whether his patients did well. I could see that he and Dr. Layan respected each other immensely and worked well together. I trusted him completely.

Robbie, my radiation oncology nurse clinician, my gentle teddy bear, met with me weekly prior to my appointment with my radiation oncologist, took my weight, blood pressure, temperature, pulse, and oxygen level. We chatted about how I was doing, and he made suggestions and gave me instructions and sample products for my side effects. He came up with solutions to help my radiation burns and mucositis. He felt like a friend.

Mary, my oncology nurse clinician, was there on infusion days and saw me before I saw Dr. Fidler. She discussed questions or concerns I had about my infusions or general well-being. She watched over my blood pressure and other medical problems that I normally saw my internist for. She was concerned about my emotional state and quality of life during treatment. She was friendly and patient, taking as long to talk with me as I needed. She entered all this information into my record.

All members of the Department of Head and Neck Cancer met at weekly "Tumor Board" to discuss the best options for new patients and to review progress of patients under treatment. This brought together not only physicians from radiation and chemotherapy, surgery and research involved in my care, but their nurses and other support staff. I was reassured to know that they sat down and talked about me together, confident that nothing would be misunderstood or missed by poor communication. In addition to my doctors and nurses, present at these discussions were:

My clinical coordinator was my go-to person whenever I needed quick advice or help with the system. She did a volume of paperwork required to document my condition and care and also managed my prescriptions and suggested remedies to make me more comfortable. She got priority appointments for me with therapists or for tests when needed, sometimes multiple appointments back-to-back for my convenience. It was a great help to have someone who knew the system and saved me hours of scheduling on the phone. She also had many helpful suggestions.

Since I was receiving treatment under a study protocol, **Mandy, a clinical research nurse,** had to complete the paperwork and be sure required appointments were scheduled and kept. She helped me complete the many pages of questionnaires that would have taken hours for me to do on my own. She was another pair of eyes during all phases of treatment, ensuring that everything was done correctly and on time. She was present at many of my appointments with my doctors and added another level of care. Strict procedures were followed, and results were recorded and compared nationally for the clinical trial.

I met with **Judith, my speech pathologist,** weekly. Her knowledge, familiarity with and concern for my particular problems, and recommendations helped to strengthen the muscles that kept my throat, tongue, speech, and swallow functions operating, resulting in my completion of treatment without the need for a feeding tube.

My dietitian made sure I had adequate nutrition, which is so important for successful treatment of cancer. I also saw her weekly. Under her guidance, I didn't lose an excessive amount of weight and continued to get adequate nutrition to support the havoc that was being generated in my body during my treatment.

Although at the beginning I thought speech and nutrition specialists were excessive, as therapy went on, I realized that they were teaching me how to go through everyday life as a cancer patient.

All these specialists were present at tumor board where they talked about my case, updated my symptoms and progress, and made decisions about my care. This coordination of care approach not only reviewed all the facts but avoided conflicting instructions and allowed each of my providers to give me the same advice.

This level of service is medicine as it should be.

The next group of angels and heroes were those who actually performed my treatments:

Oncology nurses managed the eight chemotherapy infusions I received, one each week. In the infusion room, three or four skilled chemotherapy nurses administered infusions to patients spread through the "pods." I saw the same faces each time, and these ladies became familiar during the three hours I was in the department each week. One nurse would take charge of my care at each session, but all were present and available if needed. They were all friendly, caring, competent, and treated me with respect and concern for my comfort.

Radiation therapists positioned me on the radiation table, attached my mask, and entered the data and ran the machinery that delivered the radiation program written for each day. Most of my care was delivered by three individuals. The therapists rotated so each therapist remained skilled for the variety of cancer treatments that took place in the department. I was fortunate that two in my group of three therapists were present at almost all thirty-five treatments, and I appreciated their familiar faces and caring attention. I saw Paul and Vani Monday through Friday for most of two months, and they felt like friends.

There were also **radiation physicists and dosimetrists** working behind the scenes that I never met.

Because I had been responsible for hiring and training receptionists and medical assistants during my working life, I know there is a tendency to undervalue these team members. They are often referred to as "the girl" or "the guy," implying that they are less important. Yet they are the first people patients encounter, and the way those encounters take place can make or break an impression of the visit. Dissatisfied patients generally point not to their medical care but to how the phones were answered, how quickly their registration took place, how politely they were treated when they arrived, how long they had to wait, etc. It takes very special people to create a welcoming, caring, and competent impression, especially when dealing with the sick and frightened. To undervalue their importance is a huge mistake.

I'm happy to say that the staff at Rush met this challenge.

The **reception staff** in both oncology and radiation therapy made me feel welcome, signed me in, verified my identity and appointment details, printed and processed my paperwork, attached my ID bracelet, and gave me a parking sticker and directions— all efficiently, courteously, and with a smile. They knew their work was not as simple as pressing buttons and saying "next."

Since weekly blood tests were required to monitor my condition and be sure no dangerous levels would interfere with treatment, a **phlebotomist** took my blood prior to each oncology visit and infusion. Invariably they were cheerful, chatty, and competent people. I never had to be "poked" more than once, and bruising was rare and minimal.

Medical assistants escorted me to the examination room and took my blood pressure, temperature, weight, oxygen level, brought up my file on a computer screen, and entered the values obtained. Although I knew it was far from the truth, there is a tendency to blame the medical assistant when the wait in the exam room is longer than desired. Like most people, what I wanted was not to talk to an assistant, but to see my doctor and get on with it. It takes a caring and patient person to remain positive while treating cancer patients, especially since sick people may be irritable.

Identification checks are a routine part of the process. At each step along the way, every time I saw a new member of my team, I was asked to verify my name and birthdate, my ID bracelet was checked, the information was matched to "stickers" that were attached to my paperwork and blood collection tubes, and computer entries were made.

The number of people involved in treating cancer is astounding. It's no wonder that the cost of medical care is so high, with all the salaries that must be paid. I must have identified over twenty-five Angels and Heroes by now.

In addition to traditional cancer treatment, integrative help is available for cancer patients having difficulty handling anxiety, pain, fatigue, side effects, or those who just want to be more in control of their health.

Fortunately, I was more than happy with the support I got from my medical team, my family, and my friends. It was reassuring to know, though, that other options existed. Some, but not all, of the resources were offered at Rush. I was given a list with contact information at my first oncology appointment. I could pick up literature about a variety of support groups and organizations from racks in reception rooms as well. It seemed that no matter what a patient might need, someone out there provided it.

Services offered were:
Integrative and behavioral medicine complements:
- Acupuncture
- Biofeedback
- Guided imagery
- Herbal counseling
- Individual counseling
- Massage therapy
- Medical hypnosis
- Pharmacists
- Yoga

Non-medical support:
- Social workers
- Financial counseling
- Palliative care
- American Cancer Society
- Community psychosocial and support services (List of specific support and educational groups available to handle emotional aspects of cancer treatment in a range of community settings.)

Post-therapy providers:

Throughout the years that followed cancer treatment, some of my providers moved on and were replaced by others to continue following my care and manage late effects. Key among these was **Dr. Al-Khudari,** who became my ENT when Dr. Thomas retired. It was hard to imagine anyone who could follow in Dr. Thomas's footsteps, but Dr. Al-Khudari truly is that person. He is a young, slender man, skilled in his field, whose friendly questions make me know at every visit that he really cares about me not only as a patient, but as a person.

Similarly, when Dr. Layan left Rush I met a new radiation oncologist, and **Ashley** and **Josh** continue my **speech therapy**.

All these people have been there to hold my hand through the late effects and help make my life as normal as possible. They have done so with their excellent medical knowledge and thorough and caring attention. They have been available to me whenever something new comes up, and always treat me with respect.

Family and friends:

I may be mentioning family and friends last, but that's not a reflection of their importance.

I don't know how I could have gotten through cancer treatment without my husband, Chris. He drove me to every appointment and waited with me, shopped for groceries or anything I needed, took over the bulk of household chores, and gave me encouragement and compliments. He never complained about our lack of social activities or his meals during treatment. He even let me pick television programs—although he kept control of the remote and I had to keep waking him up to change channels. That's the short version—you get the idea.

My sons, daughters-in-law, and grandchildren were very supportive too. They called frequently, bought me comfort items, visited when I was up to it, sent cards and gifts to cheer me up. Bob and Dolly, both doctors, were available whenever needed. My family all wanted to do more, but there really wasn't much to do. It would have been impractical, although they were willing, to involve my family in routine care on a day-to-day basis, so most of it fell on Chris.

Long-time friends Dorothy and Sue sent the Prayer Box and the cancer motivational plaque and called to cheer me.

I received many cards and emails from friends, neighbors, and organizations I belonged to: my writers' groups, the Lemont Public Library, the Lemont Historical Society, and the Downers Grove Choral Society. I received flowers and gifts. I collected my cards in one of those decorative photo boxes, and the box eventually filled to overflowing.

One friend, who had moved to Key West some time before my diagnosis, sent me a card every week.

Another friend enrolled me in an organization called "Better Every Day." The group sent encouraging messages, a comfort package that included the thermal bag I carried to the hospital every day, and even an envelope full of handwritten letters of encouragement from children.

I was enrolled in prayer societies and received prayer cards.

A high school friend I hadn't heard from in fifty years sent a card and note.

A group I had spoken to about my novels sent a card.

Readers who had followed my blog sent emails full of encouragement, prayers, and thanks. Fans of my books sent me notes that convinced me I had touched the lives of others.

Special thanks to the members of my writing critique group: Rod Brandon, Luisa Buehler, Mim Eichmann, John Payne, and Lee Williams. These talented and generous people helped me not only through the months of cancer treatment and recovery, but gave excellent opinions and advice throughout the writing of this memoir.

Many others, some strangers, offered to help in any way, but really, I was so surrounded by caring family, friends, and medical providers there was little I needed other than their notes and prayers.

When something as life-threatening as cancer occurs, it's wonderful to hear from people you care about. It makes you feel worthwhile. I often thought that when I die, the most meaningful thing to me would be for everyone who had touched my life to take a moment and think, "How sad. She was a good person and I liked her." I feel that cancer gave me an opportunity to see that in life.

God:

I'm Catholic but not a frequent churchgoer, and I don't consider myself a strongly religious person. Despite that, I turned to God throughout my treatment and recovery. His presence as a constant in my life was there, especially at the lowest points when I was fighting my own emotions. After dealing with cancer, when I was moving forward once again, I realized I emerged as a different person. Cancer is a wake-up call that leaves questions about whether one is leading the life one wants to lead. Since the potential for death is part of the experience, you ask yourself if you are prepared for death. You also ask if you are satisfied with God's place in your life. Perhaps you may wish for the faith you had as a child, before you became distracted by working your way through life. Whether or not God is a part of your life, cancer can help you put your life into perspective, if you allow yourself to answer those questions.

Angels and Heroes, I love you all. I can't thank you enough. Whether you supported me with your caring, skill, and kindness in person, on the phone, by snail mail or email, or from heaven, you mean more than I can say.

I'm going to stop now because I'm crying.

STAYING ALIVE IS A LOT OF WORK: ME AND MY CANCER

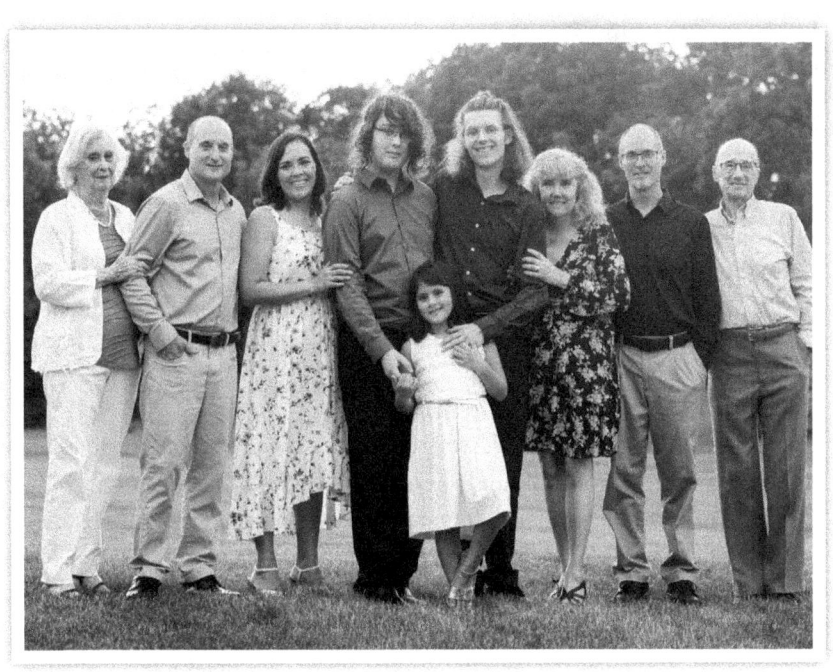

My family, 2023. Me, Bob, Dolly, Collin, Mia, Aidan, Clare, John, and Chris.

ABOUT THE AUTHOR

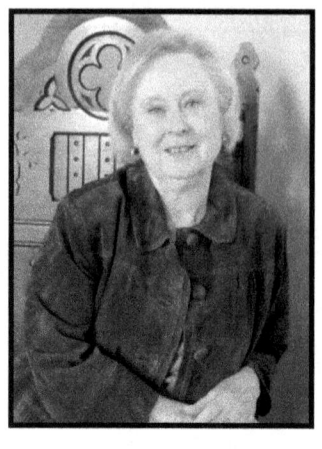

Pat Camalliere is the author of The Cora Tozzi Historical Mystery Series. Camalliere has lived in the Chicago area all her life and became intrigued by the unusual, sometimes mysterious region along the Des Plaines River Valley and Sag Valley in the Southwest suburbs of Cook, DuPage and Will Counties in the Greater Chicagoland area. Wanting to share that fascination with others, she began writing historical mysteries set in this locale, finding that a hint of the paranormal fit perfectly into the setting for the stories she wanted to tell. Her books relate a mystery from the past to a mystery in the present, while enlightening readers with details in both time periods through storytelling that surprises even lifelong residents. *Staying Alive Is a Lot of Work: Me and My Cancer* is her first memoir.

Camalliere holds a Bachelor of Arts from Saint Xavier College. She lives with her husband in Lemont, Illinois, serves on the board of the Lemont Public Library District, and oversees the archives of the Lemont Area Historical Society. She writes a blog on local history, and speaks to organizations and book clubs on a variety of topics related to local history, her cancer experience, and writing. She is a lifelong avid reader and enjoys classical choral singing. Visit her website, www.Patcamallierebooks.com, or contact her for speaking engagements, interviews, or at any time at Pat@Patcamallierebooks.com.

www.ingramcontent.com/pod-product-compliance
Lightning Source LLC
Chambersburg PA
CBHW050856160426
43194CB00011B/2172